The ICU Guide for Families

The ICU Guide for Families

Understanding Intensive Care and How You Can Support Your Loved One

Lara Goitein, MD

ROWMAN & LITTLEFIELD
Lanham • Boulder • New York • London

Published by Rowman & Littlefield
An imprint of The Rowman & Littlefield Publishing Group, Inc.
4501 Forbes Boulevard, Suite 200, Lanham, Maryland 20706
www.rowman.com

86-90 Paul Street, London EC2A 4NE, United Kingdom

British Library Cataloguing in Publication Information Available

Library of Congress Cataloging-in-Publication Data
Names: Goitein, Lara, 1969- author.
Title: The ICU guide for families : understanding intensive care and how you can
support your loved.one / Lara Goitein, MD.
Description: Lanham : Rowman & Littlefield, [2021] | Includes bibliographical
references and index. | Summary: "This book is for ICU patients' families,
suddenly immersed in an alien and intimidating world. It clearly explains intensive
care ranging from the details of the equipment and environment, to decisions
about end-of-life care, focusing on how the reader can become an effective
advocate for their loved one"— Provided by publisher.
Identifiers: LCCN 2021023122 (print) | LCCN 2021023123 (ebook) | ISBN
9781538153949 (cloth) | ISBN 9781538153956 (epub)
Subjects: LCSH: Intensive care units—Popular works. | Critical care medicine—
Popular works.
Classification: LCC RA975.5.I56 G65 2021 (print) | LCC RA975.5.I56 (ebook) |
DDC 362.17/4—dc23
LC record available at https://lccn.loc.gov/2021023122
LC ebook record available at https://lccn.loc.gov/2021023123

For Noah and Mason

Contents

List of Figures

Preface

During the twelve years I worked as an intensive care unit (ICU) physician, it became clear to me that no one in the ICU suffers as much as the family members of patients. Patients are usually sedated and mostly unaware of their critical condition. But the anguish of families is fully felt and vivid. Their world has been upended; they hang on the edge of the void.

Yet all too often family members are the forgotten souls in this drama. They sit alone in a waiting room or at the patient's bedside, hoping someone will finally come to tell them what's happening to the person they love – but doctors and nurses pass by, not stopping. When someone does finally come to talk with them, the person is often hurried and all but incomprehensible to the family. And family members may be so overwhelmed that they don't even know how to formulate their questions.

In my experience, most family members desperately need clear, straightforward explanations about intensive care and the new world they have entered, which their busy doctors and nurses don't always have time to provide. Many also feel profoundly helpless. They know that their loved one is in danger and in the hands of strangers, but they have no idea whether or how they can help.

This book is for those families. Every patient is different, but there are pressing questions and concerns that arise again and again – and I realized that I have built a repertoire of explanations that I have given over and over to family members through the years. This book is essentially a compilation of those explanations, with a focus on empowering family members to be effective advocates for their critically ill loved ones.

Now I practice outside of the ICU setting, taking care of patients with lung disease. People sometimes ask me if I "liked" practicing ICU medicine. The word is too simple to capture feelings about a profession in which many of your patients are desperately ill. What I can say is that practicing ICU medicine felt profoundly central and important. As an ICU doctor, you are regularly a part of what are the most intense and pivotal moments of peoples' lives. You know patients intimately, through immersion in their physiology. And although you may never speak to a patient, you may learn the most important and private things about them: Do they love their life? Do they believe in God? Are they ashamed of asking for help? What are they scared of? Who matters most to them and what is the mettle of those relationships, which present a clear reflection of the person? Inconsequential details, surface layers, and small talk are immediately irrelevant and fall away – and you are right in the heart of what matters. This kind of privilege doesn't exist anywhere else.

Acknowledgments

I would like to thank my three readers for their generous gifts of time and insight. I'm profoundly grateful to my brother-in-law, Jerry Hauser. His thoughtfulness and ability to empathize with imagined family members in the ICU, no doubt sharpened by his own recent experiences, were invaluable. My colleague Dr. Susan Pasnick once again proved herself one of the smartest and most knowledgeable ICU doctors I know – it is immeasurably reassuring to have had her expert eyes on this project. And last but not least, my mother, Dr. Marcia Angell, brought the same elegance, heart, intelligence, and perfect grammar with which she has edited my writing since I was five years old. Not everyone is lucky enough to have an editor-in-chief of the *New England Journal of Medicine* as a mother, and Marcia Angell, at that. I would like to thank my many mentors and teachers of ICU medicine, including Dr. Taylor Thompson, Dr. Mark Tonelli, Dr. Gordon Rubenfeld, Dr. J. Randall Curtis, and Dr. Leonard Hudson. It is amazing to see that the most interesting things being written about ICU medicine are now being written by the kids with whom I trained, including Dr. Jeremy Kahn and Dr. Catherine Lee (Terri) Hough – now they are my teachers, too. I greatly appreciate the tutelage of Ms. Wanda Jiron in issues pertaining to hospital billing. I would like to thank my wise agent, Ms. Alice Martell, and my publishing editor Ms. Suzanne Staszak-Silva. Finally, thanks to my husband, Tom Burdick. He is also a doctor, and contributed his intelligence and experience to these pages during many conversations at the dinner table. He helped me to carve out the time for this project with his typical warm generosity, good humor, and enthusiasm.

Introduction

The intensive care unit (ICU) is an intimidating place, overwhelming to most people on the outside. This book is for anyone who is suddenly immersed in this frightening world because a family member or close friend needs care there. Its purpose is to tell you in direct and simple language what you need to know to navigate this new world, and to be an effective advocate for the person you love. My hope is that a friend, doctor, or the hospital will give you the book at the beginning of your journey, and that it will come with you each day and keep you company in the ICU waiting room. I've organized the book roughly chronologically, that is, according to the time since your family member arrived in the ICU, so it addresses issues and events in the order they commonly arise. (If you got a late start, don't worry: the early chapters will still be relevant to you.) Most chapters include at least one section called "*What can you do?*" set aside in a textbox, that gives specific ideas for how you can support and be an advocate for the patient.

Even before the COVID-19 pandemic, many of us directly or indirectly had some experience with ICUs. About four million people in the United States are cared for in an ICU each year,[1] and more than a fifth of everyone who dies in the country will do so after an ICU admission.[2] Tragically, the pandemic has increased the chances that many more of us will experience ICU care. COVID-19 raises some special issues, such as visitation and infection control policies, which are discussed in chapter 5 of this book – but for the most part, the ICU experience is similar for patients with or without COVID-19.

Some parts of the book will not be relevant to all readers, and can be skipped – for example, chapter 5 which is devoted to COVID-19, and chapter 7 which is devoted to the process of dying in the ICU. In more technical sections, readers should feel free to skip to the content that is applicable to their situations. This is particularly true for chapter 4, which is devoted to surgical procedures that are common in the ICU. Throughout the book I refer to the patient at various times as your loved one, your family member, or your relative – recognizing that no one term captures all the relationships that might bring you to the bedside of someone in the ICU. To avoid the awkwardness of using multiple pronouns, I have settled on using the male gender for the patient (although of course your relative may be a woman), and the female gender for health care providers (both doctors and nurses).

This book is in no way intended to supplant the advice of your health care providers. Your ICU team will be able to give you advice and information based on the specific condition of your loved one, which I cannot do. And there is simply no substitute for a strong, trusting relationship between your family and your ICU team. This book is intended to supplement your understanding, acknowledging the reality that physicians and nurses are often unable to take the time you (and they) would like for open-ended explanations. My intention is for it to stimulate and focus important questions and conversations.

The reasons people require ICU care vary widely, as do the circumstances and the likely outcomes. But one thing is universal: having someone you love in the ICU *is likely to change you.* You will probably feel the need to be braver, stronger, more patient, more resilient, and more strategic than you have had to be throughout most of your life – and how you respond will be with you for a long time. You will remember the experience always, your memories both intensified and distorted by anxiety and sleep deprivation. If this is your first day in the waiting room, you are probably already beginning to know that disoriented, unreal feeling, as you experience the shock of your new situation.

I hope that instead of looking back on this experience as a time of being dazed and helpless, you remember it as a time in which you acquired a sense of understanding and purpose, and most importantly a feeling of pride that you were able to be the best possible advocate for your family member. An ICU stay is never a good thing, but it can be a time of increased family closeness and clarity about what is most important. You will have a lot of time to process today's shock and disorientation in the future – but right now, you have an important job to do: to be fully there for the person who needs you.

As you begin this journey, take heart. Your loved one may seem impossibly ill. But the ICU is designed to take care of the sickest of the sick, bringing all possible expertise and resources to bear – *and the large majority of its patients survive and get better.*

1

The First 24 Hours

WAITING

Why are you in the waiting room? Why can't you see your loved one? Why isn't anyone telling you anything? These are questions that intensify with every passing minute.

During the first several hours after a patient is brought to the ICU, the doctors and nurses are usually fully occupied "stabilizing" the patient. That means attaching monitoring devices, doing urgent medical procedures, and starting treatments necessary to rescue the patient from the immediate danger that made ICU care necessary in the first place. Someone may come to ask you a few brief, targeted questions about the patient – for example about prior illnesses or their medications – but this person may or may not be the doctor in charge, and may or may not take time to explain the situation to you. She might be needed at your relative's bedside – or might still be collecting information, so isn't yet ready to answer your questions.

As an ICU physician, I tried to speak with family members as soon as possible – say, within the first hour after admission – even if only briefly. I knew family members were desperate for information. If I got there quickly, I could address their concerns and establish a trusting, working relationship. If I was too late, I would sometimes find them distrustful, or even angry. But getting to the family within the first hour isn't always possible. Not only does your relative need to be stabilized, but there may be other patients admitted to the ICU simultaneously who also need stabilization.

Generally speaking, a patient is considered to be stabilized when the oxygen levels in his blood, his heart rate, and his blood pressure are consistently in a safe range. Once that is achieved, everyone can take a deep breath, step back, and take more time for reflection and discussion. The doctor responsible for your relative's care can then speak with you at more length.

Be aware that during this waiting time, when you are tremendously vulnerable and dependent on your relative's doctors, you are prone to have strong reactions toward them based on initial impressions: resentment and distrust, at one extreme, to unquestioning adulation, at the other. In most cases, neither reaction is wholly appropriate. Remember that the doctors are very likely busily working on behalf of your loved one, and there will be time for discussion and explanation after stabilization. Most caregivers know how important you are to the patient's story and ultimate outcome.

What can you do?

During waiting, contact family members and your relative's primary care physician, if he has one. Ask someone to bring you a blank notebook that you can use to keep notes. Review the events of the days leading up to the ICU admission and consider writing them down to help solidify your memory. Ask someone to bring in the patient's medication list or, even better, the actual medication containers. Try to find – or ask someone else in the family to find – medical records, test results, and advance directives (which may name someone to make decisions for the patient if necessary, or may specify the patient's wishes about treatment at the end of life). Try to remember any medication allergies your loved one has. This is all information that will be useful to the ICU doctor when she finally has a chance to sit down with you and talk in detail.

WHO ARE ALL THESE PEOPLE, AND WHO IS IN CHARGE?

Medicine, and particularly ICU care, has become so complex that care is generally provided by a team of people, each with a different area of expertise. To make things more complicated, ICU caregivers work in shifts, and the person in each specialty area will periodically change. A section called "The ICU Team" in chapter 2 goes into detail about the different people who are likely to play a part on the caregiver team. However, at this point what you should know is that there *is* one person who is designated to be in charge at any given time. This person is formally called "the attending physician" or the "attending of record" – or colloquially, "the ICU doctor." This is the person who should have the best understanding of the whole picture, and directs the care given by the team.

A notable exception is that in some teaching hospitals, residents or fellows (doctors undergoing specialty training after medical school) are given considerable autonomy in providing care – albeit under the supervision of the attending physician. If you are in a teaching hospital, a resident or fellow is likely assigned to your relative. (If you're not sure whether you are in a teaching hospital, the easiest way to find out is to ask the ICU secretary or one of the nurses, "Do you have resident physicians training here?") *Often these trainees will know the details of a patient's condition and the daily plan even better than the attending physician, and will serve as your most useful point of communication with the team.* This sounds worrying, but remember that residents and fellows have had their medical degrees for years: there is no other profession in which people are supervised so long and closely after obtaining their degree. Compared with attending physicians, some of whom spend most of their time in outpatient settings or research labs, residents and fellows spend more of their day immersed in hospital care of very sick patients, and often have more recent, intensive experience with many technical procedures. At the Massachusetts General Hospital, where I trained, if I were a patient in need of ICU care, I would rather have a senior resident perform most procedures than the average attending physician.

Another crucial point of contact for you will be the ICU nurse assigned to your relative. She will be the most readily accessible person to you, and highly knowledgeable in terms of the minute-to-minute details. She will also be in close communication with the doctors and can help you to make contact with them when necessary.

What can you do?

When you arrive at the ICU, ask your relative's nurse for the name of the attending of record (the head of the team). If it is a teaching hospital, also ask for the name of the resident or fellow with primary responsibility for your relative. You should have the opportunity to speak with one of these people within a few hours after admission (in a teaching hospital you may not meet the attending of record until the morning after a night-time admission). If you feel uncomfortable with the care being provided or the information you are being given, you have the right to ask to speak with the attending of record. For example, you might say to the nurse, "I know that everyone is very busy, but I would really appreciate a chance to get an update from the doctor, when she is available. Could you let her know? I will be in the waiting room for at least the next hour and a half."

WHO IS GOING TO BE THE MEDICAL DECISION-MAKER?

Often patients in the ICU are not able to make and communicate their own decisions – for example, when they are deeply sedated or unconscious. Someone must make decisions for them. Who should that be? Many people assume that will be the doctor in charge. That is true of certain straightforward decisions. But some of the most important decisions depend on the patient's values and preferences. Except in emergencies, these decisions require consultation with someone, optimally chosen earlier by the patient, and usually a family member. Many people have prepared documents called "advance directives for health care," for example "living wills." These usually name a proxy – also sometimes called a medical decision-maker – who has the authority to make health decisions when the patient cannot. Advance directives may also specify treatments people either want or don't want, such as dialysis in case of kidney failure.

If there is no advance directive naming a health care proxy, each state has a default system for identifying a decision-maker. These vary slightly, but typically, the proxy will be the person who comes highest on this list:

1. Legal guardian (e.g., parent of a minor, or legal guardian of someone with a disability)
2. Spouse (if not legally separated) or domestic partner
3. Adult son or daughter (eighteen or older)
4. Parent
5. Adult brother or sister
6. Close adult friend

In general, it is best if the proxy keeps close family and friends informed and involved in decisions. Doing so from the beginning can help provide the proxy with support, and also prevent miscommunication and hard feelings. But it is also important that everyone clearly understands and respects who the proxy is, whether through specific designation by the patient or through default assignment by state rules.

What can you do?

If you are the medical proxy, tell your relative's doctor and nurse. If there is a document specifying that to be the case, bring it in (or have someone else bring it) at your first convenience, to be copied and placed in the patient's chart. Explain to the nurse that when you are not there, even if there are other visitors present, you would like to be informed of important developments. Let your relative's other family and friends know that you are the proxy, and that you welcome their input. But be ready to put boundaries if needed on the extent to which other people participate in decisions.

This can feel like an awkward conversation. As an example, you might say, "According to [the patient's living will/state law], I'm legally Tom's proxy. Of course I'm planning to confer with you closely about decisions, but I wanted to make sure you understood my legal status and are comfortable with it. I don't want there to be any confusion, especially if decisions have to be made quickly."

"WE NEED TO GET YOUR SIGNATURE" – CONSENT AND COMMON EARLY PROCEDURES

When a doctor or nurse first comes to talk to you, they may not have time to talk at length, but may want to ask for your verbal or written consent to do something for the patient. (This is assuming the patient is unable to make or communicate his own decision.) If you are the patient's proxy, your consent must be obtained for major procedures such as surgery – but it is often also requested for smaller, more routine ICU procedures. In emergency situations, doctors are not legally required to obtain consent, so this step may occasionally be missed.

Four procedures commonly done in the first day are:

1. *Intubation:* This procedure is necessary if your family member will be placed on a mechanical ventilator to help him breathe. A thick tube called an endotracheal tube (endotracheal tube, often spoken as "E-T-tube") is inserted through your family member's mouth (or less commonly, nose) and down into the large central airway called the trachea.

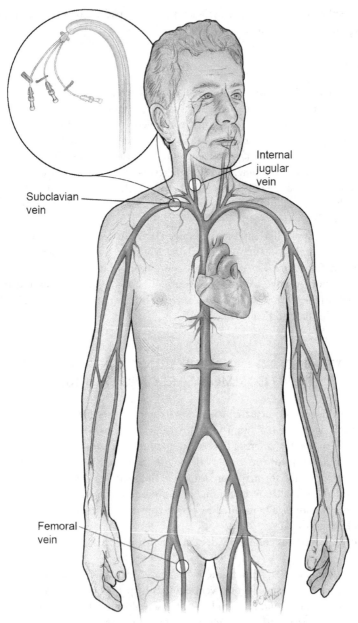

Figure 1.1. Central venous catheter and insertion sites © 2021 Laurie O'Keefe

Then the endotracheal tube is attached to the mechanical ventilator, which delivers breaths through it. Your family member will likely receive rapidly acting sedative medications before the endotracheal tube is placed. He will also likely receive a paralytic medication, to prevent motion of the muscles in the throat during the procedure; this should wear off within minutes to an hour. (See the first section in chapter 4 for more about intubation.)

2. *Insertion of a central venous catheter (or "central line"):* A central line is a flexible tube that is inserted into a large vein – usually in the neck ("jugular central line"), upper chest ("subclavian central line"), or groin ("femoral central line"). The diagram shows a central line and the three locations where it typically is inserted.

   The central line usually stays in place for a period of days, and is used for administering medications, monitoring pressures in the large veins, and drawing blood. (See the second section in chapter 4 for more about central lines.)

3. *Insertion of an arterial catheter ("a-line"):* An arterial catheter (or "a-line"), resembling a standard IV catheter, is inserted into an artery, usually in the wrist. The purpose of the a-line is to monitor pressures in the artery, which essentially provides a continuous, very accurate measurement of blood pressure. It is also useful for measuring the concentration of certain chemicals and gases in the blood. For example, an arterial blood gas (ABG) test provides important information about oxygen and carbon-dioxide levels in the arterial blood, which helps in the management and support of the patient's breathing. Arterial blood is a better measure of what vital organs are receiving than venous blood. (See the third section in chapter 4 for more about a-lines.)

4. *Blood transfusion:* Your relative may need a transfusion of blood (or components of blood, such as platelets or plasma). This is especially so if he has been admitted to the ICU because of blood loss – for example, bleeding from the stomach or intestine, or as a result of an accident – or is unable to form clots normally. (See the fourth section in chapter 4 for more about blood transfusion.)

All of these procedures are so common early in an ICU admission as to be almost routine, and although they each carry risks, *the bottom line is that you will probably want to give your consent for these procedures quickly.* In the "What can you do?" section below, I suggest just two questions to pose.

What can you do?

- If a central line is recommended, ask: "I've heard that central lines can cause bloodstream infections. Would it be possible to use a mid-line catheter instead, or would that not work in this case?" Midline catheters are a little larger than regular IVs, and like central lines can stay in place for several days – but they carry fewer risks. They cannot provide all the functions of central lines, however, so are not appropriate in every case.
- If intubation is recommended, ask: "I've heard that paralytics are often given during intubation. If you use a paralytic, please promise me that you will make sure he is completely asleep beforehand. I hate the idea of him being awake but not able to move during the procedure."

The above is a very quick discussion, designed for a busy and exhausting first day. But when you do have the time and bandwidth, you should learn more about consent and procedures, as they will probably be an ongoing part of your ICU experience. I give a fuller discussion of how to approach giving consent in chapter 2 of this book. In addition, all of chapter 4 of this book is dedicated to providing detailed descriptions of the many procedures common in the ICU, and their risks – including the four procedures described briefly above. Feel free to go to chapter 4 to read about these now, if you would like more detail.

"WE NEED TO KNOW WHAT YOUR LOVED ONE WOULD WANT" – DECISIONS ABOUT LIFE SUPPORT AND CODE STATUS

If your relative can no longer make decisions and you are the proxy, a doctor or nurse might come to ask you about "code status." A "code" is the colloquial medical term for cardiac or respiratory arrest, meaning a person's heart has stopped working effectively or he can no longer breathe on his own. Code status refers to whether and how cardiopulmonary resuscitation will be done in the event of a code.

Don't be alarmed by the question: the fact that you are being asked about "code status" does not mean that your family member is imminently at risk. It is the policy in most ICUs to establish code status for *all* patients on admission.

The options for code status are "full code," "DNR/DNI," and, less commonly, just "DNR" or "DNI."

- *Full code* – Every step will be taken to perform all aspects of cardiopulmonary resuscitation and to maintain life. The *cardio* (meaning dealing with the heart) portion of cardiopulmonary resuscitation includes electric shocks to the chest (defibrillation), chest compressions, and medications to restart and regulate the heart. The *pulmonary* (meaning dealing with the lungs) portion includes putting a breathing tube down the patient's windpipe (intubation) and attaching it to a mechanical ventilator (breathing machine).
- *DNR/DNI* – This stands for "Do Not Resuscitate/Do Not Intubate," and it means that none of the above measures will be taken. The DNR portion refers to restarting the heart, while the DNI portion refers to putting a person on mechanical ventilation. This is essentially a decision to allow a patient to die if he can no longer breathe and his heart has stopped.
- *DNR* – This stands for "Do Not Resuscitate," and means no shocks or chest compressions. Your relative could still be on a mechanical ventilator (for example to support him through an acute respiratory illness such as pneumonia).
- *DNI* – This stands for "Do Not Intubate," and means just that – the person should not be intubated and put on a mechanical ventilator. Efforts to restart the heart could still occur, but in practice they would need to be limited to a very brief attempt, as anything further would also require mechanical ventilation.

Your relative might have already completed an advance directive specifying that he would not want cardiopulmonary resuscitation, in which case the appropriate code status will likely be straightforward. Otherwise, the medical proxy will need to answer the question. If you are the proxy, this can feel like a heavy responsibility. But recognize that your job is not to decide what *you* want for your relative – but to do your best to communicate *what you think he would want* based on what you know of his values and the conversations you have had. Sometimes this requires great selflessness.

Some family members are initially mystified by the question about code status. Why on earth *wouldn't* you restart the heart and lungs? Isn't that worth at least an attempt? The reason is that the very fact of needing cardiopulmonary resuscitation means that the person is very sick: in the best-case scenario, they will likely have a long and difficult hospital course; and in the worst-case scenario, they may not survive to be discharged – or they may survive but with impaired brain function and quality of life. Some patients or proxies might reasonably feel that the risks of pursuing such care are too great, particularly in cases where the patient is very elderly or terminally ill.

While a limited code status is often lumped together as "DNR/DNI," it is important to realize that the issues for mechanical ventilation (to which "DNI" refers) and cardiac resuscitation (to which "DNR" refers) differ quite a bit. The need for intubation and a breathing machine has a very different meaning in different situations, and the outcome can be quite good (to illustrate the point, almost everyone who has minor or elective surgery is temporarily on a mechanical ventilator). Among all patients in ICUs who require a mechanical ventilator, more than two-thirds survive.[1]

In contrast, the need for cardiac resuscitation has a worse prognosis (likely outcome), and only about a fifth of patients who require cardiac resuscitation in the hospital survive to discharge – and that figure is much lower for patients who are elderly or ill with chronic disease, such as cancer.[2] Cardiac arrest means that the heart is not pumping well and that blood and oxygen are not being sufficiently delivered to the rest of the body. This can lead to damage to vital organs such as the kidneys and brain. For those who survive cardiac arrest who are older than 65, more than half have moderate to severe neurological disability at the time of discharge, many of whom must be discharged to a nursing facility or hospice rather than home.[3] The major risk of successful cardiac resuscitation, then, is that you will save the patient's life, but he will not be the person he was.

Unfortunately, the media have given us a false impression of the chances of success with cardiopulmonary resuscitation. Usually it's depicted in a young, otherwise healthy (and often beautiful) person. A doctor or bystander thumps on the chest a couple of times, and the patient wakes up utterly restored. Particularly for the elderly or those with chronic illnesses, it seldom works out that way.

The other consideration which often seems to make a big difference in decision-making is that chest compressions must be forceful and electric shocks powerful – broken ribs and skin burns are common, and there are sometimes injuries to the spine or to internal organs. When considered as an abstract concept, family members may want to do everything possible despite small chances – but they may change their minds when confronted with an understanding of how violent resuscitation actually is.

Deciding in advance whether to resuscitate a patient if he has stopped breathing or whose heart has stopped beating is complex – like other end-of-life decisions. It depends on the character and beliefs of the person, and the specific details of the health situation and likely outcome. But you often don't have the luxury of considering all of that in the first day in the ICU. The doctors and nurses might still be in a stage of information-gathering, and they might not even have a firm diagnosis yet – let alone know what the ICU course will hold. The most important information will probably be forthcoming over the next 24–48 hours. Whether your loved one will begin to round the corner in that time is a crucial piece of information that no one has at this point.

My starting bias is that, *unless there are clear arguments against cardiopulmonary resuscitation (discussed below)*, your loved one should be "full code" in these first 24 hours while the ultimate outcome is likely to be uncertain. After the first day or two the picture will begin to clear, you will have time for a thorough discussion with the doctor, and you can make more informed, less pressured decisions. The patient or the proxy always has the right to withdraw medical care – so if your relative is placed on life support, that life support can be removed. (In that case, your relative will be given medication to keep him comfortable during the dying process. This is discussed further in the section "A comfortable death" in chapter 7.) In fact, many proxies make the conscious decision to permit life support for a predefined period (e.g., three days), and then revisit the decision.

But there are cases in which it would make more sense for the patient or proxy to choose DNR/DNI code status right away, without waiting for more information. What would be some reasons to do so?

1. Your relative has an advance directive that specifies no mechanical ventilation or cardiopulmonary resuscitation, or has otherwise communicated clearly that he/she would not want such measures.
2. A doctor whom you trust tells you that your relative's condition is irreversible and cardiopulmonary resuscitation is close to hopeless.
3. Your relative is very elderly or has a serious illness such as metastatic cancer or liver failure, in which case the chance of survival with a meaningful quality of life after cardiopulmonary arrest is small.
4. Your relative has already undergone repeated cardiopulmonary resuscitation today.
5. Your relative, for whatever reason, has been consistently ready to let go. Many people who are very elderly or chronically ill have made their peace with the idea of the end. This is no failure – to the contrary, it shows courage and dignity. It is important to distinguish whether your loved one is ready to let go from whether *you* are ready to let him go. He may be ready long before you are, and your job is to represent his wishes, not yours.

What is a "short code"?

A "short code" is cardiopulmonary resuscitation that is attempted, but abandoned if the patient does not respond in a short time. This is a controversial term, and a controversial topic. On the one hand, it makes sense: a longer duration of cardiopulmonary resuscitation means more time that the body's organs are not receiving optimal blood flow, a higher chance of damage to organs, and a lower chance of survival. So especially for older people or others whose chances are less favorable, it might make sense to make an initial attempt, but give up before there is substantial risk of bringing the person back in a permanently damaged state. On the other hand, there is no firm cut-off time that predicts a bad outcome, and many doctors find it cleaner and less morally complex to think of resuscitation as "all or nothing," "black or white."

In my opinion, it is our obligation as doctors to consider the shades of gray. For patients who are full code and who are young and healthy, I favor very intensive and extended attempts at resuscitation. For patients who are classified as full code but are very elderly or are in poor health at baseline, I favor a shorter duration of resuscitation, to minimize the possibility of bringing the patient back to a life they would not reasonably want. In my experience, many doctors, whether consciously or subconsciously, do the same.

Would you want to be present during cardiopulmonary resuscitation?

There is an increasing trend to invite families to be present during cardiopulmonary resuscitation. It is thought that this might help family members to understand that everything possible to bring the patient back to life was implemented, and, if the resuscitation is unsuccessful, to grasp the reality of death and say final goodbyes. There is some data to suggest that family members present during cardiopulmonary resuscitation have less psychological distress than those who are not present.[4] However, as described above, cardiopulmonary resuscitation is by necessity violent, and it is very hard to watch your loved one in that situation. The bedside is crowded with busy people and equipment, so there is no real opportunity to provide meaningful contact or comfort to your loved one.

People have very different feelings about this. Personally, if it were my family member, I would not want to be present. If resuscitation were not successful, I would not want those to be my last images of my loved one. You should come to a decision about this, as there will be no time to deliberate if cardiopulmonary resuscitation is needed. Be ready to say either, "I would like to stay during the code, if you are OK with it," or "I'm going to leave the room now."

What can you do (if you are the proxy and the patient cannot make his own decisions)?

- Obtain and consult your relative's written advance directive if it exists.
- Recognize that your job is to represent your best understanding of what your relative would want, not what you (or others) want.
- Ask the doctor directly if she believes your relative's condition is reversible, or whether cardiopulmonary resuscitation is nearly futile.
- If you decide that your relative will be "full code," consider setting a time to reevaluate with the doctors and other people close to the patient. In 72 hours, say, your relative's prognosis (probable outcome) will likely be clearer.
- If you decide that your relative will be "full code," consider telling the doctor that you think your relative would not want a *prolonged* resuscitation attempt.
- Remember that there are many situations in which it would be reasonable to allow intubation and mechanical ventilation if necessary, but to decline cardiac resuscitation. Ask your doctor whether your relative's situation might be one of those.
- Involve close family members and friends in the discussion and in conversations with the doctor. But if you are the health care proxy, make it clear that you will at some point close the discussion and take full responsibility for the final decision. They will likely be grateful not to carry that responsibility themselves.
- Decide ahead of time whether you would want to be present during cardiopulmonary resuscitation, in the event (however unlikely) that it occurs.

BEING IN THE ICU ROOM

Interacting with your loved one

Finally, a caregiver (likely a nurse) has come to tell you that you may come to see your loved one.

He is likely surrounded by an overwhelming and confusing array of machines and monitors, with multiple tubes and wires attached to his body. Monitors might be flashing and beeping intermittently. One or more people will probably be busy in the room, moving about his bed, working at a computer, and adjusting equipment.

Do not allow yourself to be alienated or distanced from your loved one by all this equipment and activity, or by fear of being "in the way." He is still very much the same person and has never needed you more. You belong right next to him, at the head of the bed (unless a caregiver temporarily needs to be there to do a task). You may talk to him and hold his hand, even if it is strapped down to the bed or to a board. Unless you are unusually rough or clumsy, you will not dislodge any important tubes or lines, which should be firmly taped in place. Ask the nurse if you may pull up a chair to the bedside.

Your relative is likely to be drowsy or asleep, either because of sedative medications or because of chemical or other physiological changes that occur with critical illness. If so, can he understand you, or register that you are there? No one can know for sure. In my opinion, it is best to assume that he can hear you, is aware of your presence, and can derive comfort from the sound of your voice. Talk to your relative as if he were fully conscious. Identify yourself and explain what is going on, even if you might think he should already know: It's Maggie, I love you, you are in the hospital, you've been here since last night, you had a heart attack but are getting better, your children are on their way, your dog is being walked by the neighbor, your nurse's name is Mary and she's really nice. Many ICU patients suffer from anxiety and confusion – sometimes hallucinations and delusions – because of the disorienting environment and their illness. Most of them need soothing, orienting conversation, a familiar voice, and someone holding their hand. This is something extremely important that you can do for the person you love.

What can you do?

- Recognize that it is still your loved one underneath all that machinery and tubing.
- Go to the bedside and hold his hand. Ask the nurse if you may pull up a chair.
- Even if the patient seems to be asleep, talk to him as if he is awake.
- Be soothing and help orient the patient to where he is, what day and time it is, and what is happening.
- If your relative wears hearing aids, ask the nurse if they can be used.

Lines, tubes, wires, and machines

Now that you have taken your rightful place by your loved one's side, it's time to introduce you to all the lines (small tubes or catheters), tubes, wires, and machinery. For your reference, I've provided an illustration of the ICU patient and room, labeled with letters corresponding to descriptions below.

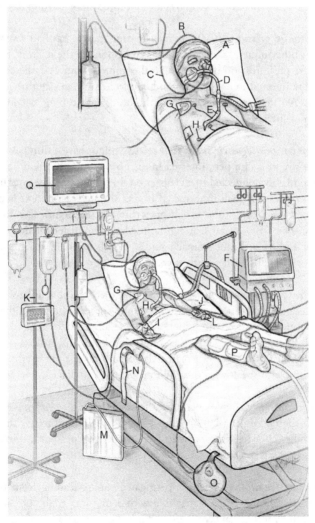

Figure 1.2.   Lines, tubes, wires, and machines: The equipment in the room © 2021 Laurie O'Keefe

Don't feel the need to learn all this now – you can come back to this section and identify equipment as you are curious, or when questions arise.

A. *Tape over the eyes:* When patients are receiving sedatives or have swelling around their eyes, their eyes may not fully close when they are sleeping. You might see tape holding your relative's eyes closed, and his eyelids might be shiny with ointment. These measures are to protect his eyes from drying.

B. *Intracranial pressure (ICP) monitor:* If your relative has had severe brain trauma or other injury, he may have this to help guide the doctors' therapies to optimize pressures and blood flow to the injured brain. A catheter or wire is surgically inserted into the brain and connected to a device that monitors pressures. You may see a bandage over the head, with tubing extending to a bedside measurement device.

C. *Nasogastric or orogastric tube:* Your relative might have a thin plastic tube, about the size of a slim pen, inserted in his nose or mouth, the other end of which is probably connected to a canister on the wall. This tube goes into the patient's stomach or small intestine. If it goes through the nose it is called a nasogastric tube ("N-G-tube"); if it goes through the mouth it is called an orogastric tube ("O-G-tube"). It can be used to administer medications and nutrition, and to suck out stomach juices, blood, or air in the stomach. It should not in itself interfere with speech.

D. *Endotracheal tube:* If your relative needs a mechanical ventilator, he will have an endotracheal tube inserted in his mouth (or less commonly, the nose). It ends up in the trachea (windpipe), a few inches below the vocal cords. See chapter 2, figure 2.1, to see how the endotracheal tube sits in the airway. The tube is secured to the face by a plastic device and tape. Your family member will not be able to speak with the endotracheal tube in place.

E. *Suction catheter:* Often a suction catheter, sheathed in plastic, is left connected to the endotracheal tube. This can be fed down through the endotracheal tube, allowing intermittent deep suctioning of sputum and other secretions in the airways.

F. *Mechanical ventilator:* There is corrugated tubing leading from the end of the endotracheal tube to a machine with a monitor at the bedside. The machine is the mechanical ventilator, and it is doing some or all of the work of breathing for the patient. The air being delivered is humidified, so there may be some water collecting in the tubing between the patient and the mechanical ventilator. Ventilators are described in more detail in the section "The breathing machine" in chapter 2.

G. Central line: Your relative might have a bandage over his neck or upper chest, with 2–4 thin protruding tubes. The bandage covers the insertion site of a central venous catheter, or "central line," which is a large IV inserted into one of the major veins of the neck or chest (or, less frequently, the groin). Central lines were discussed earlier in this chapter, and typical insertion sites were shown in figure 1.1. If the central line was inserted recently, there may be some blood on the bandage (which will probably be changed soon). The protruding tubes are used to administer intravenous medications and fluids, and to draw blood samples. The central line is also sometimes used to measure pressure in the large veins (called central venous pressure, or CVP), which can give the doctors important information. Some central lines can be used for hemodialysis or to insert a pacemaker if the heart rhythm is abnormal.

H. ECG electrodes and leads: Your relative probably has small adhesive pads on his chest, connected to wires or "leads." These are connected to a heart monitor, which displays a continuous electrocardiogram (ECG).

I. Arterial catheter: There is either an arterial catheter ("a-line") for invasive blood pressure monitoring (usually in the wrist, but sometimes in the upper arm or groin), or a blood pressure cuff on the arm for "noninvasive blood pressure" (NIBP) monitoring. If your relative has a wrist a-line, the wrist may be strapped to a board to hold it in position. The a-line is connected to tubing that extends to a device called a pressure transducer, which measures the blood pressure. Pressure readings are taken continuously and displayed as a pulsating line on the overhead monitor that shows vital signs. In contrast, NIBP recordings are taken intermittently: at a set interval, you will hear a humming noise, the blood pressure cuff will tighten, and a new blood pressure reading will appear on the monitor.

J. Intravenous catheter (IV): Your relative might have one or more IVs in the arm to administer medications and fluids.

K. IV pole: One or several IV poles will stand next to the bed, to which pumps (to administer medications), pressure transducers, and other equipment are attached. Bags of medications and fluids are hung on these poles.

L. *Oximeter:* Your relative probably has a device to measure oxygen saturation clipped or taped to his finger. It measures how much oxygen the blood is carrying. Sometimes, if the skin or blood flow in the fingers makes it hard to get an accurate reading of oxygen saturation, an oximeter will be clipped or taped to the earlobe, forehead, or toe.

M. *Chest tube and atrium:* Your relative may have a chest tube, which is inserted between the ribs to drain air or fluid from around the lung. You will see a bandage across the chest, and thick tubing extending from under the bandage down to a rectangular collection box, called an atrium, which sits or hangs below the bed.

N. *Restraints:* There may be cushioned straps around the wrists and/or ankles, tied to the rails of the bed. These are designed to prevent the patient from pulling out lines or tubes when he is asleep or confused.

O. *Urinary catheter:* There might be a urinary catheter (a common type is a "Foley catheter") inserted through the patient's urethra into the bladder, with urine flowing into a collection bag that hangs down below the bed. The bag must always stay below the level of the pelvis to allow drainage in the correct direction. Some catheters are attached externally, rather than actually inserted into the urethra – for example, "condom catheters" for men.

P. *Sequential compression devices (SCDs):* Often called "pneumoboots," these are intended to prevent blood clots from forming in the veins by intermittently squeezing the legs to promote blood flow. While the stockings are inflating, you will hear a mechanical noise from the air pump.

Q. *Vital signs monitor:* The large monitor to show vital signs is a screen mounted overhead to allow clear visualization at all times. Some of the information commonly shown on the monitor display is listed here and depicted in figure 1.3.

Typical ranges are given below for each measurement; these do not represent "normal" values, but values commonly seen in sick ICU patients.

- A continuously running electrocardiogram (ECG) showing the electrical pattern of the heartbeat.
- Blood pressure, shown as a ratio of systolic blood pressure (usually 85–170) to diastolic blood pressure (usually 40–95). If there is an a-line

Electrocardiogram (ECG) tracing

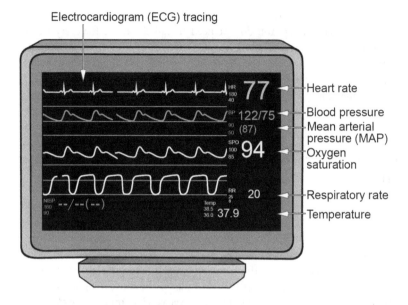

Figure 1.3. Vital signs monitor © 2021 Laurie O'Keefe

there will be continuous readings of blood pressures, as shown in the figure.

- A number showing mean arterial pressure (MAP), often in parentheses and next to the blood pressure (usually 60–85 in ICU patients). This is a slightly different way of providing information about blood pressure.
- A number representing heart rate (HR; usually in the range of 50–135 beats per minute in ICU patients).
- A number showing oxygen saturation (SpO2; usually in the range of 85–100% in ICU patients).
- A number showing respiratory rate (RR; usually in the range of 8–30 breaths per minute in ICU patients).
- A number showing body temperature, often in degrees Celsius (usually 36.0–39.5C in ICU patients).

Responding to alarms in the room

Monitors are usually set to sound an alarm when measurements are outside the normal range. The problem is that particularly in the early hours of admission, when stabilization is still underway, measurements are *often* outside the normal range (usually falling somewhere in the wider ranges I provided in the previous section). Alarms frequently sound when nothing dangerous or important is happening. You do not need to call the nurse for every alarm. Important measurements are usually projected onto a screen somewhere in the central nursing areas outside the room. Rest assured that at least one person is keeping an eye on them, even when the patient's nurse is out of the room. If the measurement is worrying, a nurse will respond soon.

That being said, "alarm fatigue" – a condition in which nurses and other staff start to tune out and ignore alarms because there are so many of them – is a real problem. Rarely, a family member plays an important role in bringing attention to an important measurement more quickly than would otherwise happen.

What can you do?

Some family members of ICU patients quite happily ignore the numbers on the monitors and the alarms – and that is just fine. Others are very interested in learning what the numbers mean and keeping track of them. If you are the latter type of person, how do you strike the right balance between concern, on the one hand, and overreacting, on the other?

I suggest that for the first day, while you are getting used to what the numbers mean and their patterns, you try to ignore the frequent alarms and abnormal values, and trust the doctors and nurses to respond appropriately. As you get more familiar with the measurements, you will have a better sense of what is truly unusual. As a rough guide, if a number jumps suddenly to a very different value, you should consider calling the nurse. For example, if the heart rate has been in the 80s or 90s for the day, and suddenly jumps to 150, the nurse should be promptly informed. If there is a slow creep that eventually triggers the alarm, you can generally wait until the nurse is next in the room.

COMMON MANIFESTATIONS OF ILLNESS IN THE ICU

By and large, medical problems in the ICU can be thought of in three categories: the primary illness that triggered the admission, the secondary manifestations of critical illness, and the complications that may arise over time (usually after several days in the ICU). Figure 1.4 shows this schematic, and important examples in each category.

There are many causes of critical illness that bring patients to the ICU in the first place (the primary critical illness). Some of the most common

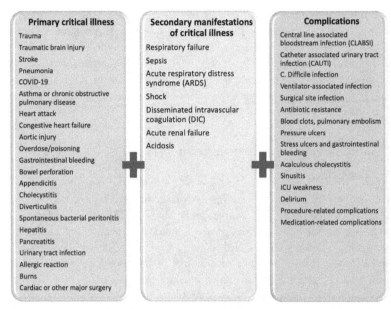

Figure 1.4. Categories of medical problems in the ICU. Courtesy of the author

include infections (for example, pneumonia from pneumococcus, influenza, COVID-19, or other microbes), a heart attack or heart failure, trauma such as motor vehicle accidents, gastrointestinal bleeding, bowel perforation, stroke, pancreatitis, and overdoses of alcohol or other drugs. It's beyond the scope of this book to go into detail about all the illnesses that can bring a person to the ICU. Instead, this section deals with the handful of common *secondary* manifestations of critical illness: the common ways in which the body responds to many different kinds of injury. While some ICU care will be directed to your relative's primary illness, much of ICU care will target the common secondary manifestations. You are likely to hear some of the terms for these conditions from nurses and doctors, and this section is meant to help you understand them. This is a technical section – you may wish to read only about the terms you have heard applied to your relative at this time, and perhaps come back to other terms later if needed.

For more explanation of the primary cause of your loved one's critical illness (pneumonia, stroke, etc.), I recommend the source *UpToDate* (https://www.uptodate.com). This is a comprehensive online source designed for physicians, but most of its chapters include an excellent summary designed for patients. Many hospitals provide their staff with this resource for free, so you could ask your nurse or doctor if they would be willing to print or email you the "Information for patients" section provided under the topic most relevant to your loved one's diagnosis. If you have friends who are doctors, there is also a good chance they will have access. (You could get your own subscription, but it is expensive – perhaps worthwhile though if you are anticipating complex health care needs over the coming year.) The third category of medical problems – complications – will be discussed later in this book (in the last section of chapter 3), as they tend to arise later.

Common secondary manifestations of critical illness

Respiratory failure

The primary function of breathing is "gas exchange," in which oxygen is brought into the body (via the lungs) and carbon dioxide is expelled from the body (also via the lungs). If your relative is not able to breathe well enough to carry out gas exchange, it is called respiratory failure. There are many reasons for respiratory failure, including pneumonia, an asthma attack, and congestive heart failure. Even problems that are not related to the lungs can cause respiratory failure – for example, neurologic problems that interfere with breathing. Respiratory failure that primarily affects blood levels of oxygen (for example, from pneumonia) is often called "hypoxic" respiratory failure, while respiratory failure that primarily causes the retention of carbon dioxide (for example, from asthma) is often called "ventilatory" or "hypercarbic" respiratory failure. In either case, patients with respiratory failure require assistance with breathing, either with a mechanical ventilator or with other types of support that do not require intubation – for example, bilevel positive airway pressure (BIPAP), in which pressurized air is delivered to the patient through a face mask. Ventilators and other types of support for breathing are discussed in more detail in the section "The breathing machine" in chapter 2.

Sepsis

Sepsis is a severe infection accompanied by a very strong immune response – so strong that it causes problems with normal organ function. The infection can arise from any source – for example, pneumonia, a urinary tract infection, or appendicitis. In some cases, the original source of infection is never identified. Often, but not always, bacteria from the infection is found in the blood ("bacteremia"). Sepsis can cause illness ranging from mild to very severe, so the outcome varies widely. In severe cases, intense inflammation throughout the body can lead to low blood pressure and shock (see below), kidney failure, blood clotting abnormalities, liver failure, acute respiratory distress syndrome (ARDS, see below), and other organ damage.

Shock

Shock is a very serious, critical condition which may result from many causes (including sepsis). It means that there is inadequate delivery of oxygen to the tissues of the body, resulting in organ damage. It almost always occurs in the setting of very low blood pressure. Shock may result from:

1. Heart failure with inadequate pumping of blood ("cardiogenic shock"); for example, from a massive heart attack.
2. Inadequate volume of blood; for example, from heavy bleeding ("hemorrhagic shock") or severe dehydration.
3. Leakiness and/or dilation of blood vessels; for example, from infection ("septic shock"), a severe allergic reaction ("anaphylactic shock"), injury to the brain or spinal cord ("neurogenic shock"), or certain poisonings.

Your ICU team must work fast to correct the underlying cause of shock, while supporting the ability of the lungs and circulatory system to deliver oxygen more effectively.

Acute Respiratory Distress Syndrome (ARDS)

ARDS is an inflammatory process in the lungs that affects about 1 in 10 patients admitted to ICUs. Causes include severe infection, whether in the lungs (such as COVID-19 or a bacterial pneumonia) or elsewhere in the body; trauma (such as from a motor vehicle accident); severe burns; injury to the pancreas; and drugs and toxins. ARDS often occurs with sepsis. To meet the definition of ARDS, a patient must have (among other things) very low blood oxygen levels and chest X-rays that show widespread abnormalities throughout both lungs. Most patients with ARDS have respiratory failure and require mechanical ventilation. There is no specific treatment for ARDS other than time, and treating the underlying condition. However, it is particularly important in ARDS to avoid using mechanical ventilation settings that inflate the patient's lungs with too much air. That creates further injury to the lungs in patients with ARDS, and smaller breath sizes have been shown to be associated with a much better chance of survival. For this reason, you may hear that your relative is receiving "low tidal volume ventilation" (LTVV), "lung-protective ventilation," or "ARDS-protocol ventilation."

DIC (Disseminated Intravascular Coagulation)

DIC is abnormal clotting in the blood, leading to both overactive blood clotting and abnormal bleeding. It can cause destruction of red blood cells and organ failure. A patient with severe DIC may develop bruising and dark spots on his or her skin, and bluish fingers and toes. Like sepsis and ARDS, DIC is a reaction of the body to many different types of injury. These include severe infection, trauma, metastatic cancer, burns, certain complications of pregnancy, and rarely, severe reactions to transfusion.

Acute Kidney Injury (AKI) – also known as Acute Renal Failure (ARF)

These interchangeable terms refer to a rapidly developing inability of the kidneys to function normally. There are multiple causes. A common one is poor oxygen delivery to the kidneys – usually in the setting of low blood pressure or overwhelming infection. Other causes include toxicity from certain medications (such as the dye used in certain imaging scans), obstruction of urine flow (for example, by a tumor or kidney stone), poisoning, obstruction of the blood vessels leading to the kidneys, and autoimmune diseases. More than half of ICU patients develop at least some degree of AKI.

The kidneys perform an important role in excreting just the right balance of chemicals and fluid from the body. When the kidneys are injured, urine production may decrease. Certain chemicals such as potassium, acid, and urea can accumulate in the blood and reach unsafe levels. Because of the decrease in urine production, fluid might back up into the rest of the body and lungs, causing swelling and shortness of breath. The patient might require dialysis to help remove fluid and certain chemicals. In the ICU, this is usually done with hemodialysis, in which the patient's blood is pumped through a machine (via a large central line) to do some of the work of the kidneys. Hemodialysis is discussed in more detail in chapter 4.

Often, AKI in the ICU is fully reversible and lasts only a few days. However, it can be prolonged and require weeks or months of dialysis. Most people who previously had normal kidney function will eventually no longer need dialysis, although kidney function may never return completely to normal.

Acidosis

Acidosis refers to a low blood pH, which is a measure of how much acid is in the blood. Normal arterial blood pH is 7.35–7.45. When pH is lower than normal, the blood is too acidic, and the patient is said to have acidosis. This is common in the ICU and can happen for many reasons. One of the most important is lactic acidosis – lactic acid accumulates in the blood because of the effects of massive inflammation, shock, liver failure, widespread metastatic cancer, or certain drugs and toxins. Acidosis provides information about the underlying illness and its severity, but usually does not in itself require treatment. If acidosis is extreme, however, it can cause heart failure, low blood pressure, and shock. Methods of treating acidosis include increasing the rate or volume of ventilator breaths to get rid of carbon dioxide, giving bicarbonate (a base which counteracts the acid), and, if necessary, dialysis.

TAKING CARE OF YOU

You have survived the first 24 hours. I hope you have now had a chance to talk at length with your loved one's doctors and gain an understanding of what happened and what treatments have been initiated. You are probably exhausted. But you have accompanied your loved one through the most hectic and dangerous part of an ICU admission.

You may have been so preoccupied during this day that you have forgotten to eat, drink, sleep, or even go to the bathroom. This is understandable – but it is simply not sustainable. At this point you need to start thinking of this experience as a marathon, not a sprint, and begin to pace yourself. You will need to take care of your own biological and psychological needs, in order to be the best advocate and companion you can be for your loved one.

Ask the nurse or doctor whether your loved one is stable enough that it is safe for you to leave the ICU without missing important changes or decisions. If so, and if you have other family or friends with you, ask them to take a shift staying in the ICU to allow you to go home to get some sleep and a shower – and maybe a walk for some fresh air. Tell the nurse and your family and friends that you want to be called immediately if there is any change in your loved one's condition. Your family and friends will want very much to help – but may not be sure how. Asking them directly to do things like take a spell for you in the ICU, pick up food, or run errands will likely be a relief for them.

If you are like many family members of ICU patients, you have spent much of the first day wondering if you could have done anything differently to avoid this crisis: "I should have insisted that he check his blood sugars more often!" "Why did I let that ER doctor send him home on Sunday instead of admitting him to the hospital?" "If I hadn't gone to the movies, he wouldn't have been alone at home and fallen." You may also have been spending much of the day bargaining with God or the universe: "If you only let him get better, I promise I will . . ."

It's time to put those thoughts aside. You simply do not have the energy to spare to punish yourself. You need to be kind and protective of yourself, so that you can be fully present for your family member – who is going to need you. And who loves you.

So put down this book and – if you can – go home and get a little bit of well-earned rest.

2

The First 3 Days

You've gotten through the first day and, hopefully, your loved one has stabilized to some extent. It is now time to develop more familiarity with your new environment – the people, the concepts, and the equipment.

This time period is an important one. The first 2–3 days provide time to stabilize the patient, and to begin treatment for the underlying problem that brought him to the ICU in the first place. Whether your loved one is beginning to turn the corner after this initial period of care carries important information about what his ultimate course will be. Even for patients who are initially very sick, showing improvement within the first 48 hours means the average chance of survival is close to 95 percent – much better than for patients who stay the same or get worse over the first 48 hours.[1]

THE ICU TEAM

If you are older, you may still remember when care was given primarily by one doctor and a nurse. But in the past several decades, medical care – particularly in the ICU – has become so complicated that most patients now require a whole team of people, each with a different role and expertise. The good news is that your relative will benefit from having many experts involved in his care. The downside is that communication can be challenging – it can sometimes feel like it isn't clear who is in charge, and that no one person is taking responsibility. (Remember, at any given time there will be an attending physician for your relative: *this* is the person with final responsibility. If you are not sure who that is, ask your nurse.) Probably you have already met a large number of people involved in taking care of your family member, who may or may not have identified themselves to you. The following are typical members of an ICU team.

Attending physician

This is the doctor with ultimate responsibility. She is in charge of directing care and coordinating the team. In an ICU, the attending physician is likely a physician specializing in lung and ICU care (pulmonary and critical care medicine), but alternatively she could be a cardiologist, anesthesiologist, surgeon, or internist. Other staff may refer to her as "the ICU doctor." What is confusing is that the attending physician position rotates – attending physicians tend to work in 12- or 24-hour shifts. Often the same attending physician will take the day shift for several days or even weeks in a row, to allow for some continuity of care. This will be the doctor who knows your loved one best – but when she is "off," she is "off," and another doctor steps in. Whichever attending physician is currently on call is the "boss," and you should speak with the boss for a periodic update or if you have intervening concerns about care. The attending physician may or may not be supervising a nurse practitioner or physician's assistant. The size of the role taken by nurse practitioners and physician's assistants varies widely (some are very proficient and manage many of the details of day-to-day care).

Trainees: Medical students, residents, and fellows

If you are in a teaching hospital, young doctors at various stages in their training may be helping to care for your relative. *Medical students* do not yet have their medical degrees and are spending time working on hospital teams as part of their education – they are typically closely supervised. *Residents* do have their medical degrees. A residency is somewhere between work and school. On the one hand, residents are paid (albeit not well) and are relied on to do much of the work of patient care in the hospital. On the other hand, they are also being trained in a specialty of medicine (for example, internal medicine or surgery) and are supervised by an attending physician. First-year residents are often called "interns." *Fellows* have completed a residency, and are subspecializing further (for example, after my 3-year residency in internal medicine I completed a 3-year fellowship in pulmonary and critical care). In some of the best teaching hospitals, residents and fellows are given considerable autonomy and are responsible for directing care – albeit under the supervision of the attending physician. Often they will know the details of the patient and the daily plan even better than the attending, and will serve as the most useful point of communication with the team. To summarize, the hierarchy from top to bottom is: attending physician → fellow → resident → intern (a first-year resident) → medical student.

ICU nurse

A nurse will be assigned to your relative during each shift (usually 12-hour day and night shifts). Your relative may be the only patient assigned to that nurse, or there may be others – but generally ICU nurses do not have more than 3 patients. The nurse is the one who will spend much of the day in the room and be the first contact for minute-to-minute needs. She is responsible for bedside care such as administering the medications and other treatments ordered by physicians, closely monitoring the patient, inserting urinary catheters and cleaning and turning the patient, and communicating as necessary with the doctors and other team members. Unfortunately nurses also have responsibility for ever more exhaustive documentation, so the nurse may be facing a computer monitor for much of the day. She may or may not have a nursing assistant or technician to help her.

Nurse manager

The ICU is generally managed by a senior nurse whose responsibilities are primarily administrative. However, the best ICU nurse managers are often out of their offices and in the patient care areas of the ICU – checking in with nurses and families, lending a hand when things are busy, and making sure that everything is going well. If you have questions about how the ICU is running, and particularly about nursing care, you should ask to speak with the nurse manager. For example, you could say something like, "I asked to meet with you to check in, and to tell you how impressed I am with how your ICU seems to run overall. I also wanted to get your advice about one concern."

Consultants

Your attending physician may ask for a consultation from a health care provider from a different medical or surgical specialty. For example, if the attending physician is worried about bleeding from the gastrointestinal tract, she may consult a gastroenterologist. If your relative develops acute kidney injury, she may consult a nephrologist. If your relative develops acute appendicitis, she may consult a surgeon. It is not uncommon for several consultants to be involved in the care of one ICU patient. Often, a consultant will have significant input and importance to your patient's care. However, she does not hold final responsibility: that belongs to the attending physician. The attending physician is responsible for coordinating the care from the different consultants and overseeing the big picture.

Respiratory therapist

The respiratory therapist is responsible for many aspects of care involving breathing. If your relative is on a mechanical ventilator, the respiratory therapist adjusts the settings according to the orders from the doctor, draws arterial blood to measure blood gases (oxygen and carbon dioxide) and pH, and may make recommendations to the doctor for changes to the ventilator settings. She will often help manage the ventilator while your relative is being transported to other parts of the hospital (for example, for radiology studies), or moved for exercise. The respiratory therapist also delivers breathing treatments and inhaled medications, and uses a catheter to suction sputum out of the airways.

Nutritionist

The nutritionist is responsible for overseeing your relative's nutritional intake. Many patients in the ICU are not able to chew and swallow food, and instead receive nutrition intravenously or through a tube that passes into their stomach (usually through the nose or mouth, but sometimes directly through an incision in the abdominal wall). The nutritionist keeps track of the calories, electrolytes, and other nutrients that are being provided, to make sure the right amount and balance are maintained for each patient.

Physical therapist

A physical therapist may be asked to recommend and oversee a program of physical activity for your family member, especially if your relative has certain special needs (for example, after a brain or spine injury).

Speech therapist

A speech therapist may be asked to evaluate and treat problems with speaking and swallowing, particularly in patients who have had a stroke, been on a mechanical ventilator, or have a tracheostomy.

Case manager/social worker

This person helps to manage logistics such as financial issues, working with health insurers, tracking down medical decision-makers and other family members, obtaining equipment and services, and planning care after your relative is discharged from the hospital. For example, she can help with matters such as Family Medical Leave Act (FMLA) forms, letters to employers, short-term disability forms, get-out-of-jail/jury duty forms, travel insurance, and arranging for housing and meals near the hospital.

Palliative care

Palliative care is a subspecialty of medicine; both physicians and nurses may have palliative care training. People often assume that palliative care exclusively focuses on end-of-life care (for example, if and when to withdraw life support). However, palliative care physicians and nurses also manage severe symptoms (for example, pain, shortness of breath, and itching). If a palliative care provider arrives to talk with you, it does not mean that the team is giving up on treating your relative! In fact, sometimes the palliative care service is routinely involved in the care of all ICU patients. It can only help to have a team member focused on your loved one's comfort and big picture goals. If you would like to talk with a palliative care nurse or doctor about either end-of-life decisions or symptom management, you should tell your family member's nurse.

Phlebotomists

If a blood sample is needed for laboratory testing, it may be collected by the nurse, but may also be collected by a laboratory technician called a phlebotomist.

Radiology technicians

These people run the X-ray, ultrasound, CT scan, and other equipment used to take images of your relative's body. Although many of them are quite knowledgeable, it is important to understand that they are not trained to interpret the studies – the images are reviewed and interpreted elsewhere by radiologists.

What can you do?

As you can see, there is a large group of people taking care of your loved one. Because they are focused on their work (and often in a hurry), they may or may not introduce themselves clearly. *You have the right to ask every person who enters the room for his or her name and role.* If a person identifies herself as a doctor, ask her to clarify whether she is a resident, fellow, or attending doctor. For example: "There are so many people coming and going. Do you mind telling me your name and your role, and what it is that you do?" If a person says that she is "from" a certain service – for example, "from the nephrology service" – ask what her specific role is (e.g., doctor, nurse, technician).

Especially for physicians (attendings, residents, fellows, and consultants), I would advise you to write down names and roles to help you to keep track. Many ICU rooms have a whiteboard on the wall with essential information about the patient and the day's schedule; if there is room, you can ask your nurse whether this is an acceptable place to write the names of the physicians with a dry erase marker. Earlier, I suggested that you keep a notebook during your relative's ICU stay – this would also be a good place to record names.

THE ICU SCHEDULE AND WHEN TO ASK QUESTIONS

Intensive care is hard, fast-paced work. In all but the sleepiest ICUs, doctors range from busy to *extremely* busy. It is also unpredictable work – there can be crises that suddenly take hours. You need and have a right to hear from your doctor about your relative, but it can be very hard to find the right time to do so. Knowing your ICU's schedule can help.

All ICUs have different schedules, but there are some typical features. Generally, both the nurses and doctors will work in 12-hour shifts (sometimes doctors work in 24-hour shifts or even longer). The day shift usually starts at 6 a.m. or 7 a.m. At this time, the night nurse will meet with the day nurse coming on duty, to pass along information about the patient (often called the "shift report"). Increasingly, shift report is being done at the patient's bedside

– and if it happens during visitor hours it provides a time for listening and questions from families. Many ICUs hold nurse "huddles" early in the morning, in which all the nurses meet in a central area to talk about assignments for the day and other practical information. These are not generally open to families (and do not provide much information about individual patients).

ICU doctors often "pre-round" on their patients, by themselves, first thing in the morning. A lot of this work takes place at a computer, for example, reviewing lab results and X-rays; however, many doctors will quickly stop by the ICU room to examine the patient and check in with the nurse. Often, this is a rushed time for the physicians, and probably not the best time for complicated questions or discussion (unless it is a visiting consultant physician, in which case it may be your only chance that day).

After the nurses and physicians on the day shift have had a chance to get caught up on their patients, many ICUs hold multidisciplinary ICU rounds, generally in mid- to late morning. Many members of the ICU team are likely to be present: doctors, doctors-in-training, nurses, respiratory therapists, physical therapists, nutritionists, palliative care, case managers and social workers. This large group – sometimes consisting of 10–20 people! – moves from room to room like a flotilla, usually rolling computers along with the group to check and enter information. Outside each patient's room, one person (in a teaching hospital, this is often a medical student or resident) will present the patient and the plans for the day and ask for input from the various people on the team. You will usually be welcome to stand with them and listen. Especially in a teaching hospital, this can be a very structured, formal presentation. If you listen carefully, you will hear that presentations follow a consistent format – by convention, something like the following:

1. Quick statement of who the patient is and why they are there
2. Major events of the past 24 hours
3. Vital signs and physical exam
4. Current medications
5. Important lab, imaging, and test results
6. Assessment and plan: What the presenter thinks about the patient's status, and what she intends to do about it that day. In the ICU the assessment and plan is often given by organ system – for example, pulmonary (lungs), cardiac (heart), gastrointestinal (stomach and intestines), and so forth.
7. Sometimes: Review of a checklist of good ICU "housekeeping" (e.g., what lines and tubes are in place and if they can be discontinued, and nutritional intake)

Multidisciplinary rounds are working rounds and are not tailored for visitors. They are businesslike and full of technical jargon, and can be intimidating to many visitors. However, families often find them useful as they provide a chance to see the whole team, and to get at least a sense of what the doctors are thinking and planning for the day. There will not be much time for questions, but after the flotilla moves on, you can ask your nurse to clarify the things you have heard. You may want to have your notebook with you during multidisciplinary rounds, to jot down information and questions.

After multidisciplinary rounds, nurses and doctors settle in to doing the work that has been planned. For example, they will send patients to get radiology studies, do procedures, give medications, call colleagues for consultation, and write notes in the patients' charts. Throughout the day, they may also be admitting new patients to the ICU from the emergency room or elsewhere in the hospital. Generally, the best time for doctors to have discussions with family members is in the afternoon, after they have completed morning rounds and gotten some of the most pressing work of the day squared away (of course, this window can disappear if a crisis arises). The evening nurses and doctors arrive around 6 p.m. or 7 p.m., and the schedule repeats itself (except that multidisciplinary rounds are usually held only during the day shift).

What should your expectations be for frequency of communication? There are no hard and fast rules. Your nurse should be readily available and often in your family member's room, and she will be able to answer questions throughout the day. During times when your family member is unstable or things are changing rapidly, it is reasonable to expect the ICU doctor (or, if it's a teaching hospital, the resident) to give you an update at least every few hours. If your loved one is relatively stable, it is reasonable to expect touching base with the doctor once a day.

What can you do?

- Remember that although the doctors are busy, you have a right to explanations. Being informed is necessary for you to support and be a good advocate for your loved one. Even if they seem rushed or impatient, doctors *do* understand this, and often feel guilty that they can't spend more time with you. Be considerate of the doctors' time, but make sure you get what you need.
- Assign one person to be the main contact person for the doctor, and responsible for passing the information on to the rest of the family.

This is much more efficient for the doctor than trying to speak with everybody, and avoids mixed messages and holes in communication for family members. In general, the contact person should be the medical proxy, but sometimes there is a doctor or other health care professional in the family who steps into this role. Make sure the contact person's phone number is prominently available in the patient's room or on his chart.

- If nurses meet at the bedside to report to each other between nursing shifts (called "shift report"), try to be there if visiting hours permit. It's a good time to get information and ask a few questions.
- Ask your nurse what time the ICU holds multidisciplinary rounds and try to be there to listen and learn the plans for the day. You can come out of the room to stand quietly with the group in the hallway so you can hear well. Remember however that these are busy working rounds, and the doctor leading rounds may or may not take time to talk with you – any in-depth conversation is best deferred until later. After multidisciplinary rounds, you can ask your nurse questions about what you heard. Keep a notebook with you during rounds to jot down information and questions.
- The unpredictability of ICU work means that doctors are never in full control of their schedules (that fact alone is a constant source of stress for them). Rather than ask the doctor to meet with you at a *specific* time (for example 2 p.m.), ask the nurse to tell the doctor that you would like to speak with her that day, and that you will be around and available during a certain time range (for example, 1–4 p.m.). You can ask the nurse whether there is a time of day that is generally better than others for the doctor to speak with you. Try to be present during that time period if possible.
- After your loved one has been stabilized, ask the doctor directly what to expect in terms of daily communication. For example, "I know that you're incredibly busy, but of course I want to stay informed. Is it reasonable to ask for a quick update once a day? If so, when is the best general time period for this to happen? I can make sure I'm available when it's most likely to work for you."
- Sometimes, a conference with multiple family members or multiple caregivers is needed – for example, to discuss end-of-life decisions. If you think such a conference should happen, ask the ICU case manager or social worker to help schedule it.

CHANGES IN YOUR RELATIVE'S APPEARANCE

One of the most distressing aspects of this situation may be the changes you notice in your loved one's appearance. Within a day or two of critical illness, many patients look quite different. It helps to understand why these changes happen – and that they are usually temporary.

Many ICU patients require large amounts of intravenous fluids to maintain a safe blood pressure. In essence, it helps to keep the pipes full of fluid to maintain higher pressures. In addition, patients' medical conditions may cause them to have leaky blood vessels so that fluids seep out into the tissues. "Anasarca" is the term for diffuse accumulation of fluid in the body tissues. You may notice swelling of the face and limbs; if you push with a finger against the skin there may be a lasting indentation (called "pitting edema"). Sometimes the swelling may be so extreme that it causes the skin to weep droplets of clear or yellow fluid. There may be swelling of the eyelids, and even of the thin membrane covering the eyeball. The eyelid may actually roll back slightly, so that the inner lining protrudes. Often, nurses put an ointment in the eyes to protect them from drying, or even tape the eyelids shut.

Your relative's skin color may seem different. Low oxygen levels or low blood pressure can make the lips, fingers, and toes look bluish, and low blood counts can make the skin pale. If blood pressure has been very low, there may be dark areas of tissue breakdown on fingers or toes. Certain conditions can cause other skin discolorations (for example, injury to the liver can cause the skin and eyes to turn yellowish, which is called "jaundice").

Usually we moisten our own lips throughout the day. When patients are critically ill and drowsy, nurses help to keep the lips moistened with wet swabs and ointments. You can ask your nurse if you can help to do this – she will appreciate it! Despite this care, the lips can become dry and cracked. Tubes inserted into the mouth for mechanical ventilation or feeding can even cause sores, despite repositioning them periodically.

Many ICU patients have multiple bruises on their arms and legs. These are caused by frequent blood draws, as well as abnormal blood clotting because of medications, poor nutrition, or the underlying condition. Poor nutrition and certain medications (such as steroids) lead to fragility of the skin, which can cause easy tearing, particularly when tape or bandages are removed. Patients who are in bed for a long time can develop sores at the base of the spine, heels, and other pressure points – especially if they are heavily sedated or unconscious for other reasons. The nurses will try to cushion pressure points and turn the patient into a different position every couple of hours to try to prevent this.

The physical changes are not all visual. There will also be changes in the person's smell. The disinfecting soaps used in the ICU smell strongly, and although nurses do their best to keep your relative clean despite not being able to take a full shower or bath, you may notice body odor. Certain medical conditions can cause potent smells as well.

Such changes are a natural, temporary part of critical illness – but they are distressing. They are distressing in part because they are a shocking visual reminder of how ill your family member is. But I think they can also be distressing because they may cause private feelings of revulsion, precisely at the time when you most want to feel close and supportive of your loved one. Be forgiving of yourself – some squeamishness is natural and does not mean you love the person any less.

It's hard to believe, but the dramatic physical changes of critical illness are generally temporary: your relative will likely return to his old self after the critical illness has resolved.

COMMUNICATING WITH YOUR LOVED ONE

Your loved one may be deeply asleep (whether because of medications or his underlying condition) – or may be in various states of alertness. Talk to your relative, whether or not he is clearly able to understand. Remind him frequently of what has happened, the date and time, how many days he has been in the ICU, and the names of caregivers. To the extent your relative can hear you, this will help to orient him, prevent confusion and panic, and provide comfort.

Your loved one may be confused and possibly restless and agitated. It is even possible he will not recognize you. Try not to be distressed by this. Delirium is very common in the ICU for many reasons, as discussed further in the last section of chapter 3, "Complications." In the elderly, even minor infections may be enough to cause profound confusion or drowsiness. The confusion usually resolves with the critical illness. Speak quietly and calmly, and remind your loved one of where he is, how long he has been here, and what has happened.

If your loved one is awake, make sure he has glasses or hearing aids, if needed. If there is room, consider putting a calendar, clock, and photos within sight. If he is on a ventilator or otherwise unable to speak, but is alert and thinking well, bring a pad of paper and see if he can write. If not, a number of "patient communication boards" are available for purchase online. These have icons for various common requests and statements from patients, as well as the letters of the alphabet to spell out other requests. Some patients can point to icons and letters on the board to communicate. In my opinion, many of these boards are too busy and complicated for very sick, sedated patients to focus on. You could consider making your own very simple, personalized communication board, with just a few useful words and phrases on the pad. For example, you could select from the following:

- Yes
- No
- Hurts
- Short of breath
- Mouth dry
- Need suctioning
- What is your name?
- Are you a nurse or a doctor?
- When will my wife be here?
- Please ask my son to come in
- When can the breathing tube come out
- What did my tests show
- Scared
- Love you
- Tell me how you are doing/news from home

WHAT IS "SUPPORTIVE CARE"?

You may hear that your relative is receiving "supportive care." Treatment can be divided into active therapies on the one hand, and supportive care on the other. Active therapies directly treat the underlying disease or condition. Examples include antibiotics for pneumonia, or surgery for appendicitis. Supportive care means interventions that support the body's vital functions to permit time for treatment and healing.

For example, medications to support blood pressure – "vasopressors" – do not treat the underlying cause of your relative's illness. They do, however, help to keep your relative's blood pressure in a safe range to buy time for antibiotics or other active treatments to work. The mechanical ventilator is also supportive care. The ventilator does not make your relative's lungs either better or worse; it simply takes on some of the work of breathing to keep your relative's breathing in a safe range while (for example) his pneumonia heals. It is a waiting tool. Nutritional support with feeding through a tube in the stomach is also supportive; it maintains your relative's general health and immune status during the course of his illness. In fact, *most* of the work of ICU care is carefully supporting the body to buy time for it to heal.

Some, but not all, of supportive care is "life support." Life support are those therapies without which the patient would rapidly die. Usually, these are the mechanical ventilator, and devices and medications that raise blood pressure to safe levels.

THE BREATHING MACHINE

What is a mechanical ventilator?

Of all the machinery in your relative's room, the mechanical ventilator (called "the ventilator" or sometimes "the vent") is likely to loom largest – both physically and psychologically. It carries hefty symbolic importance – when people say that they would not want to live "on a machine," the ventilator is what they are referring to. Yet the ventilator generally has little effect on the course of illness, but rather is the classic example of supportive care – it is not itself a treatment. The ventilator takes some or all of the work of breathing off your relative while the lungs and the rest of the body have time to recover.

Being on a ventilator, in and of itself, has little significance in terms of "how sick" your relative is. Someone can be on a ventilator for less than a day because they require an elective surgery on their knee, for example, or because they inhaled a piece of steak and it needs to be extracted. On the other hand, severe lung disease may require prolonged ventilation – carrying a much worse prognosis (likely outcome).

Breathing serves two important functions: it brings oxygen into the lungs where it can be absorbed into the bloodstream (oxygenation); and it moves carbon dioxide out of the lungs (ventilation) which is important for keeping the acid level in the blood in a safe range. This is called "gas exchange." Usually, a ventilator is needed because a patient has pneumonia or some other disease of the lung which makes the lung too stiff for the patient to breathe effectively on his own. Alternatively, your relative may require the ventilator to take on the work of breathing while he is unconscious or has chemical abnormalities in the bloodstream that interfere with normal breathing.

How is the ventilator attached to your relative?

Usually, the mechanical ventilator is connected to a patient through a tube (endotracheal tube, or ETT; sometimes spoken as "E-T-tube") that enters the

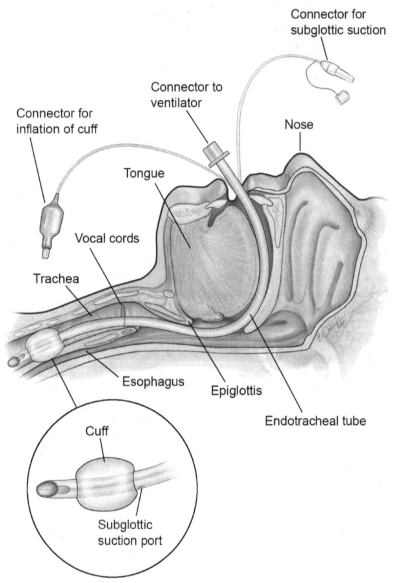

Figure 2.1.   Endotracheal tube © 2021 Laurie O'Keefe

mouth and terminates in the windpipe (trachea) a few inches below the vocal cords, as shown in figure 2.1.

A balloon (called a "cuff") near the tip of the endotracheal tube is inflated just below the vocal cords to make a seal against the walls of the trachea. Less commonly, a smaller tube can be inserted through a nostril into the trachea. If a patient requires prolonged mechanical ventilation, he may benefit from a tracheostomy, a small hole created surgically in the front of the neck through which a tracheostomy tube can be inserted into the trachea to permit mechanical ventilation. This is often done some time between 1 and 3 weeks after mechanical ventilation is started. (Tracheostomy is presented in more detail in chapter 4, and figure 4.4 in that chapter.)

Does the endotracheal tube hurt? Your loved one's throat will probably be sore for a day or so after the endotracheal tube is placed ("intubation"). Immediately after placement – and whenever the endotracheal tube is moved – it may cause gagging and discomfort. And it can take a while for the patient to relax enough to accept the ventilator breathing for him. For these reasons, initially after intubation patients often require sedation to be comfortable. But after a while, they get used to the feel of the endotracheal tube and the ventilator. Many patients are completely comfortable on the ventilator, without any sedation. Your loved one will not be able to eat normally while he is on a mechanical ventilator, and generally will not be able to speak. In rare circumstances a speaking valve can permit some limited speech even while on the mechanical ventilator, but this is usually much later.

Suctioning

You will notice that your relative's nurse or respiratory therapist will intermittently feed a tube (usually sheathed in protective plastic to keep it clean) down through the endotracheal tube – sometimes causing coughing and mild discomfort. The tube is used to suction sputum and secretions out of the airways below the tip of the endotracheal tube. You will see suctioned secretions accumulating in a suction cannister attached to the wall. Pulmonary secretions in the ICU are frequently blood-tinged for many reasons, including minor abrasions in the airways caused by the endotracheal tube and the suctioning catheter itself. Some endotracheal tubes also have a special tube that allows suctioning of secretions that pool *above* the inflatable cuff (subglottic suctioning; see figure 2.1 of the endotracheal tube, above). This helps to prevent saliva and mucus from the mouth and nose from sliding past the inflatable cuff and into the lower airway.

How does the ventilator work?

The ventilator pushes air into the lungs based on measures set by the operator (usually a respiratory therapist, working with the doctors). The concentration of oxygen in the air can be controlled. The amount of air pushed in can be controlled – either by specifying the volume or the pressure of the air delivered with each breath, as well as how often the breaths are delivered. The operator can also specify whether the ventilator will deliver all the breaths or only some of them, and whether each breath will be delivered in full or whether the ventilator will just give a little pressure to assist the breath. In this way, ventilator support can be increased or diminished to allow the patient to do less or more of the work of breathing on his own. Generally, early in the ICU admission, the ventilator controls all the breaths and assumes almost all the work. There are many different settings for how breaths are delivered (accompanied by a bewildering set of terminology), and your caregiver team will work to find the best and most comfortable one for your relative.

The above covers what most family members should know about the mechanical ventilator. But there are some family members who find it fascinating to track the actual measurements and the changes made to ventilator settings. The rest of this section is for you. Some important terms you may hear are the following:

- *FiO2* – Spoken as "ef-aye-oh-too." The fraction of inspired oxygen, which is the concentration of oxygen. It can range from 0.21 (21%, the same as room air) to 1.00 (100%). The more severe your relative's lung disease, the higher the FiO2 needed.
- *PEEP* – Positive end-expiratory pressure. After exhalation, a little bit of pressure is maintained in the breathing tube, so that the lung air sacks don't completely collapse. This helps to improve oxygenation. In general, the more severe your relative's lung disease, the higher the PEEP needed. PEEP generally ranges from 5 to 20 cm H2O.
- *Tidal volume* – The size of each breath, usually around 6–8 mL per kg of body weight.
- *Respiratory rate* – The rate at which your relative is breathing.
- *ARDS protocol* – Most ICUs have adopted a published protocol for optimal ventilator management of ARDS. This specifies small tidal volumes to avoid overinflation and injury, as well as oxygen and PEEP levels.
- *Pressure support* – This ventilator setting allows your relative to determine his breathing rate, with the ventilator delivering a specified amount of pressure to assist each breath. The amount of pressure can be turned down until the patient is doing almost all of the work of breathing, so

pressure support is commonly used when a patient is close to ready to come off the ventilator.

As a simplification, oxygenation (which increases levels of oxygen in the blood) is increased by turning up either FiO2 or PEEP. Ventilation (which lowers levels of carbon dioxide and acid in the blood) is increased by turning up either tidal volume or respiratory rate. Your relative's doctors and respiratory therapists will make adjustments to these parameters based in part on "blood gas" laboratory results.

Other kinds of breathing support

For patients with severe problems breathing, it is usually necessary to use a mechanical ventilator with an endotracheal tube. However, with less severe problems, it may be possible to help your relative with pressurized air delivered through a face mask (rather than a tube inserted into the trachea). This is called noninvasive positive pressure ventilation (NIPPV) and is usually most effective in people with exacerbations of chronic lung disease from smoking, or congestive heart failure. There are two types: CPAP (continuous positive airway pressure) and BIPAP (bilevel positive airway pressure). A patient must be conscious and alert to safely receive NIPPV – and it's not a good long-term solution. The mask must be strapped on tightly and is somewhat uncomfortable, and the pressurized air dries out the nose and mouth. But it can help to buy time when there is a cause of breathing difficulty that can be corrected relatively quickly.

Complications of ventilators

In critical illness, the ventilator is a crucial tool to support breathing – and life – while the body recovers. However, particularly if a patient is on a ventilator for a long time, there can be complications arising from the ventilator or endotracheal tube. Rarely, there can be damage to the larynx and trachea, causing bleeding, or long-term scar tissue and narrowing ("stenosis"). High pressures in the lungs can cause air to leak into the space around the lungs, sometimes causing a lung to collapse like a deflated balloon ("pneumothorax"). A more frequent complication is called ventilator-associated pneumonia (sometimes called VAP). Mechanical ventilation and some of the conditions and medications common in the ICU predispose patients to developing infections in the lungs, caused by bacteria or fungi from the hospital environment or from the patient's own gastrointestinal tract. Because these germs are contracted in the hospital, they may be resistant to common antibiotics and require powerful broad-spectrum antibiotics.

There are many things that can be done to reduce the risk of complications from the ventilator, but the most effective by far is to *get the patient off mechanical ventilation as quickly as possible – just as soon as the patient is able to breathe without assistance.* And the best way to know when this time is reached is to do frequent spontaneous breathing trials (SBTs). In an SBT, the support given by the ventilator is turned way down or off (under close monitoring), to see how your relative breathes without assistance. If your relative is also receiving sedation, it is important that the sedative medications are stopped before the SBT so that your relative is awake enough to breathe actively. This is called a "sedation vacation," or "spontaneous awakening trial" (SAT).

Without doing this testing, a patient on a ventilator who *needs* it looks very much like a patient on a ventilator who *doesn't.* A day or two can go by before the doctor realizes the ventilator can be removed – and time on a ventilator is dangerous. It's been shown that doing daily paired SBTs and SATs, to test readiness for removing the ventilator, reduces mortality rates in ICU patients.[2]

Your relative may not have an SAT/SBT in the first day or two in the ICU – there are standard reasons not to do these trials which are often present early in an ICU stay (for example, the need for very high ventilator settings to maintain oxygen levels). But as soon as possible, an SAT/SBT should be at least a daily event in order to make sure the care team is aware immediately when your relative is ready to come off the ventilator.

In addition to daily sedation vacations with SBTs, some other aspects of care that are important to preventing complications of mechanical ventilators are:

- Keeping the head of the bed elevated, to help prevent secretions and bacteria from the upper gastrointestinal tract from backing up into the throat and down past the endotracheal tube.
- Cleaning the mouth carefully at least twice a day to help cut down on bacteria.
- If the endotracheal tube has a subglottic suction port (discussed above), using it to frequently suction subglottic secretions before they can slide past the cuff into the lungs.
- Not routinely using gastric acid suppressant medications unless there is a strong reason to do so. Gastric acid suppressants allow bacteria to grow abnormally in the upper gastrointestinal tract, where they can easily move into the lungs and predispose to ventilator-associated pneumonia. These medications are indicated to prevent gastric ulcers that can develop in patients with very severe critical illness, but are probably overused.

- Encouraging mobility. Some ICU patients are so sick that it is dangerous to move them much, especially early in their ICU admission. However, most ICU patients can do some kind of activity, ranging from having their arms and legs moved and stretched by someone else (passive exercises), to doing some active arm and leg exercises, to sitting upright in bed or in a chair next to a bed. The ventilator does not in itself prevent activity – in fact, more and more ICUs actually take stable ventilated patients for walks, rolling the ventilator beside them, as shown in the illustration.

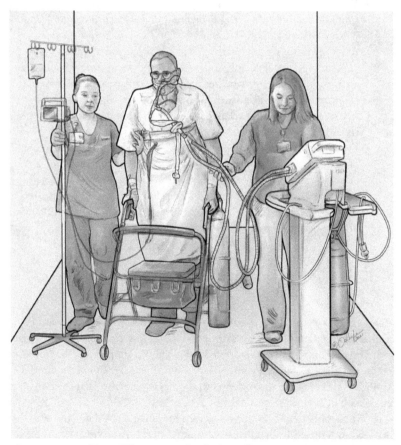

Figure 2.2. Walking while on a mechanical ventilator © 2021 Laurie O'Keefe

Programs to get patients moving earlier have been shown to decrease the length of stay in the ICU and to improve muscle strength. They may also help prevent ventilator-associated pneumonia.

What can you do?

As always, there is a balance to strike between advocating for your relative on the one hand, and not annoying caregivers on the other. The balance will differ with each nurse and doctor, and you will need to feel this out as you go. As you are able:

- Every day, ask your nurse or respiratory therapist about whether a spontaneous breathing trial is planned or has been done, and how your relative did on the last one.
- Ask your nurse if your relative is on "GI prophylaxis" with a gastric acid suppressant. If so, ask to speak with the doctor to ask if there is a strong indication, or whether it could be replaced with a non-acid suppressing medication (such as sucralfate).
- If you notice that your relative is lying flat, ask whether the head of the bed could be elevated.
- Every day, ask the nurse if it would be safe to get your relative out of bed into a chair. Also ask if you could be of help in doing passive or active exercises with your relative. ICU nurses know this is good for patients, but in practice are often too busy to spend much time assisting exercises themselves. The nurse can show you how to help, or even better, ask the ICU physical therapist to show you.

NUTRITION

Many patients in the ICU are unable to eat, usually because they are on a mechanical ventilator or are not alert. Food is of tremendous biological, social, and symbolic importance. We use food not only to support our bodies, but to connect with people and demonstrate love. After a day or two in the ICU, family members may be disconcerted to suddenly remember that their relative hasn't yet had anything to eat.

It isn't possible to go without water for more than a few days, and water is provided to most critically ill patients intravenously. However, it's possible to live without food for weeks. Despite this, most ICUs will start feeding patients a nutritional drink through a feeding tube within the first 2–3 days of admission – this is called "early enteral nutrition" or "tube feeds." ("Enteral" refers to intestines.) It's thought that early enteral nutrition may reduce the rate of certain complications – including pneumonia and bleeding from stress ulcers in the stomach – and possibly even reduce the chance of death. The published evidence supporting early enteral feeding is not very conclusive, but it's a frequent practice anyway (perhaps food is of just as much social and symbolic importance to doctors as to others). Some patients will not be able to tolerate as much enteral feeding as would be nutritionally ideal – for example, if it causes vomiting. But even for those patients, every attempt is made to provide a small amount, sometimes called "trickle feeding." It's thought that for the first week or two, the amount is not as important as just the fact of providing some protective coating and stimulation to the stomach and intestines.

Some patients are not able to tolerate enteral nutrition at all, either because of problems with their gastrointestinal tract or extremely low blood pressure. These patients can have parenteral nutrition – that is, nutrition provided through a vein. However, parenteral nutrition comes with a risk of certain infections, so it is usually not considered until 1–2 weeks after admission, when the effects of malnutrition start to become important.

Often, a nutritionist is asked to help the ICU team to calculate the type and amount of nutrition that is administered, either enterally or parenterally. If the nutrition is given enterally, it is administered through a tube that passes through either the mouth or nose into the stomach. If it is given parenterally, it is administered through a central line (an IV with the tip in a large central vein). Occasionally, if enteral nutrition will be needed for a long time, a tube (called a "gastrostomy tube") is surgically placed through the abdomen directly into the stomach. Gastrostomy tubes are discussed in more detail in the last section of chapter 4. Tube feeds are usually started slowly, and gradually advanced "to goal," which means to the calculated target rate. It is common to have some diarrhea with tube feeds.

You may hear the term "residual." This is the amount of tube feed that accumulates in the stomach during tube feeding (it can be directly measured by sucking the fluid back into a syringe). It used to be that large residuals were considered evidence of the patient not digesting well, and in response nurses would turn down the rate of tube feeding. However, this was shown not to be helpful, and is no longer done routinely.

It's hard to get used to the idea of your loved one not eating regular food, but it takes a long time to develop serious malnutrition, so try not to be too concerned. Reassure yourself that when you get home, you can cook him his favorite meal every day.

What can you do?

- On day 2 or 3 of admission, if your relative is still not receiving enteral feeding, ask your nurse or doctor whether this is a possibility.
- If your relative has started tube feeds, ask the nurse from time to time whether tube feeds are "at goal," or still at a slower rate.

CONVERSATIONS ABOUT PROCEDURES AND GIVING CONSENT

If you are the proxy, you may have already experienced the process of giving consent for a treatment or procedure. In my experience, obtaining informed consent is often done in a cursory fashion. But consent should be taken seriously and obtained only after the patient or proxy is fully informed.

If you are the proxy and your loved one is unable to give consent himself, what exactly is your role? Your goal is to make sure the procedure or treatment is consistent with what you think your relative would want. Of course, you are probably not able to evaluate the medical reasons – nor if they are worth the risks. Your doctor is far more qualified to do this, and to a large extent you will be dependent on her recommendation. But occasionally, a conversation during the consent process can change the doctor's mind about whether she recommends a procedure or treatment.

Before I wrote this section, my husband and I had a long conversation about the times we remembered changing our minds during such conversations with patients and families (he is an interventional radiologist, who does procedures all day long). The reasons generally fall into two categories. First, we have changed our minds when we were on the fence about a procedure to begin with. Perhaps we were not quite sure it was absolutely necessary but thought we should at least offer it. When families express questions and concerns about risks, doctors who are on the fence may be pushed to the other side. The second category is when patients remind us of big picture goals that may be contrary to the procedure. For example, a patient who is entering hospice may reasonably choose not to have a feeding tube placed.

So, rather than evaluate the medical risks and benefits yourself, your real goal during a conversation with the doctor is to encourage *her* to take a few moments of consideration and reflection.

In order to both inform yourself and encourage thoughtfulness in the doctor, I suggest following the mnemonic "ROTEG." See table 2.1 for an explanation of the mnemonic, and some examples of language you might use.

Table 2.1. Conversations about Consent for Procedures

ROTEG Steps		Sample language
R	Reasons, Risks, Repeat	Reasons: "Could you clarify for me what exactly you hope to learn or do with this procedure, and how it might make my family member better?"
		Risks: "What are the risks and how frequently do they occur? Does my family member have any problems that make him/her particularly high risk?"
		Repeat: "Could I please repeat that back to you to make sure I have it right?"
O	Options	"Are there any other ways to learn or accomplish the same thing?"
		"Could we first give other options a try for a day or two, or is it better to move quickly?"
T	Technique	"Who will actually be doing the procedure?"
		"I hope you don't mind me asking: How much experience do you personally have with this procedure?"
		"Do you feel like you're the best and most experienced person to do this procedure? I trust you, which is why I'm asking you directly."
		(Any questions specific to the procedure: See suggestions in chapter 4)
E	Enthusiasm	"Are you on the fence at all about whether this procedure is indicated, Doctor?"
		"If it were your family member, would you recommend this procedure?"
G	Goals	For certain patients: "We would like to give intensive care a try, but my family member has been clear that the quality of his/her remaining life is more important than quantity. Do you think doing this fits with his/her goals?"

What can you do if you are the proxy giving consent (because your loved one can't make his own decisions)?

- The consent form is standard, legalistic, and generally does not provide much information about specific procedures, so don't spend a lot of time trying to decipher it. Instead, ask the caregiver who brought you the form to explain the procedure in detail, including its risks and their likelihood. Consider using the ROTEG mnemonic described in table 2.1 to guide your discussion.

- The "Repeat" step of ROTEG is especially important. After your questions have been answered, tell the person obtaining consent that you would like to *repeat back to them what you have learned*, to make sure that you understand well. Then and only then should you give your consent for a procedure (unless it is an emergency).
- Ask your doctor, "Would you recommend this procedure if it was your own family member?"
- If the person obtaining consent is unable to answer your questions, do not hesitate to ask to speak with someone with more knowledge of the procedure.
- If severe injury or death are presented as risks, this may be just a legal "cover-your-butt" move. Make sure you really understand the likelihood. For example, you could say: "Severe injury or death sounds pretty scary. Can you give me a sense of the actual likelihood? Are these risks very rare, or a real possibility here?"
- Read about specific procedures and their risks in chapter 4 of this book.

ARE WE IN THE RIGHT PLACE? TRANSFERRING TO ANOTHER HOSPITAL

It's natural to wonder if your relative's doctors and the hospital are good enough. You have the right to ask for a transfer to another hospital, and such transfers are not uncommon – approximately 1 in 20 critically ill patients are transferred from one hospital to another,[3] for a host of reasons – including family preference, physician comfort level, and availability of needed services.

The question is: Is transferring to another hospital more likely to help or hurt your relative? There are real risks to transporting critically ill patients. For some patients with severe lung disease, even small changes in position can cause dangerous drops in blood oxygen, and moving from stretcher to stretcher in the course of the transfer is risky. In addition, moving ICU patients always carries the risks of dislodging important equipment (for example, the endotracheal tube), which can cause sudden crises. Each transfer between sending hospitals, paramedic crews, and receiving hospitals risks miscommunication, lost information, and error. In fact, more than 1 in 15 critically ill patients transferring from one hospital to another experience some type of adverse medical event during the transfer.[4]

Large urban teaching hospitals are often assumed to be the best hospitals. These hospitals have the advantage of highly specialized experts, who see rare cases that are referred from around the country and the globe. So wouldn't it be worth the risks to get to the "best" hospital? Not always. For common conditions, most smaller community hospitals are perfectly able to provide gold-standard care – and compared to large, complex medical centers, they may be easier to navigate, have a calmer pace, and provide better communication and more personal attention. However, it is probably true that if your relative has a rare or difficult-to-diagnose condition, or a condition that requires a highly specialized procedure or surgery, he would benefit from being in an academic or specialized medical center.

Unfortunately, it is also true that ICUs in some hospitals provide sloppy or poor care – no matter what the size, type, or reputation of the hospital. For example, one factor that is strongly associated with patients' survival is the nurse-to-patient ratio. ICUs in which nurses care for only one or two patients have better survival rates than those in which nurses care for three or more.[5] It's important not to be too rigid about this rule – sometimes it is appropriate for a nurse to care for three patients at once, for example, if the patients are relatively healthy, or as a temporary bridge while staffing is redistributed. But in general, if you notice your relative's ICU nurses are often taking care of more than two patients (particularly if they are all on mechanical ventilators), that is a warning sign.

There are multiple hospital grading systems available online to help give patients a sense of their quality. The best known are the Centers for Medicare and Medicaid (CMS) Hospital Compare Star Rating (ranging from 1 to 5 stars; found at Medicare.gov, https://www.medicare.gov/care-compare), and the Leapfrog Hospital Safety Grade (ranging from F to A; found at Leapfrog-group.org, https://www.hospitalsafetygrade.org). While consistently low ratings are likely a real warning sign, in my opinion you should not otherwise put too much importance on publicly reported ratings. It is well known that rating the quality of a hospital is challenging to say the least, and results are hard to interpret because of differences in things like the severity of illness and complexity of the patients that hospitals tend to see. Academic medical centers, which take care of very sick and complex patients, tend to have worse performance on public ratings as a result.[6] Ratings can also be significantly inflated by careful attention to how certain conditions are documented, and other types of gaming the system. When I see a hospital with straight "5-Star" and "A" ratings, I know immediately that they put a lot of resources into meticulous documentation; I am less certain that they truly provide better care.

What can you do?

- If your relative poses a diagnostic dilemma, has a very rare condition, or requires a procedure or surgery that is rarely performed, you may be best served in a large teaching hospital or specialized center.
- Ask your doctor directly if she thinks the hospital is the best place to take care of your relative. This is a very reasonable question, and because it is about the capability of the system (rather than the competence of the doctor), it should not cause offense or defensiveness. For example, you could ask: "I really don't have much familiarity with this hospital. Do you think that it is a good place to take care of someone in my relative's condition? Or would it be better for my loved one to be transferred somewhere else? I trust your judgment."
- If you have a family member or friend who is a doctor, it may help to have her call the ICU doctor to get a sense of the facility's capabilities.
- The following are warning signs which, in aggregate, might push you toward considering transfer:
  - Nurses often take care of more than 2 patients (especially worrisome if more than 2 of them are on ventilators).
  - On any given day, there is no dedicated ICU doctor (instead, various doctors follow patients wherever they may go in the hospital, including the ICU).
  - Your relative has been there for 48 hours and no one is yet able to tell you the diagnosis – in other words, the specific *cause* of the critical illness. Remember that sepsis, ARDS, and respiratory failure are manifestations of critical illness – not causes.
  - The nurse is unable to immediately identify the attending of record for your relative.
  - One caregiver criticizes the competence or care given by another. (This is often a response to anxiety, and likely speaks worse of the criticizing clinician than the one being criticized.)
  - The team of caregivers does not round together daily on ICU patients.
  - Your relative is frequently completely asleep and unarousable because of sedative medications (not because of his underlying condition).

- If your relative is on a mechanical ventilator, there is no attempt to do a daily spontaneous breathing trial (test of removing ventilator support), and your nurse or doctor can't give a specific reason why.
- Doctors and nurses seem too rushed to pay attention to details.
- Doctors and nurses are frequently defensive or resistant to your questions.
- The hospital consistently receives low CMS Star Ratings (1–2 Stars) and Leapfrog Safety Scores (D or F).

If you are seriously considering a transfer, speak with the case manager or social worker about costs and insurance coverage. Often insurers will cover the cost of transfer, but sometimes will require documentation of medical necessity, or will cover transfer costs only as far as the nearest facility that can provide the needed services. You should know ahead of time what you're getting into.

3

The First 2 Weeks

As hard as it is to believe, after the first few days, you are probably getting used to the routines of your strange new world. As you enter the second week, you may be moving away from crisis mode to settling in for the long term. As the adrenaline fades a little, exhaustion and doubts can hit hard: Why *hasn't* your loved one gotten well enough to leave the ICU yet? Is something going wrong?

You should know that if your relative has improved during the ICU stay so far, the chances of survival are excellent. If your relative has stayed the same or worsened, then you may be in for a longer, more difficult ICU stay – but it's important to understand that *even patients who don't turn the corner early are more likely to survive than not.* This is a time for patience, and for giving your loved one the time he needs to heal after the initial crisis. For your relative's ICU team, this is also a time of transition: from a focus on diagnosis and stabilization, to avoiding complications and providing meticulous supportive care.

INTERACTING WITH CAREGIVERS

The first sections of chapter 1 described the people likely to be involved in your family member's team of caregivers, and gave some ideas for when to ask questions of busy nurses and physicians. This section goes into more depth about the complicated social world to which, like it or not, you now belong.

In this section, I will be talking a lot about the perceptions and needs of your caregivers. You may well ask, "Why are we talking about *their* needs? My family member is the one who is sick, after all." You're absolutely correct: his needs come foremost, and most of your doctors and nurses understand that very well. As a generalization, doctors and nurses are among the most caring, tough, and resilient people I know – but they work in a high-stress, challenging environment, and they are human. Understanding their perspectives is useful to help you navigate your loved one's ICU stay.

Your relationship with your family member's caregivers is one-sided in the extreme. Not only do they have far more knowledge than you of the world that you are sharing, but they have a tremendous amount of authority – power over the one thing that probably matters most to you right now: your loved one's life. Understandably, family members may worry about whether the physicians and nurses "like" them, believing that if they can make a good personal connection it will lead to extra effort and better care for their loved one. Family members may be loath to interrupt obviously busy doctors and nurses with questions for fear of being annoying. On the other hand, family members need those questions answered, and recognize that they must advocate on behalf of the patient when things don't seem to be going right. How on earth will you walk the line between being agreeable and being a strong advocate? Is it possible to do both?

Being an advocate

It is not only possible to be an advocate for your family member: it is essential. This is in fact your most important job right now. Regardless of the competence and diligence of your caretakers, you will know certain things about your loved one that they cannot – for example, symptoms over the days before hospitalization, medical history, habits and behaviors, and beliefs and values that may be important to health care decisions. Also, in some ways you will have a more detailed understanding of your family member's hospital course. The nurse may be taking care of 2–3 patients and the doctor may be taking care of 15–30 patients at any one time. By now, they have probably rotated on and off duty in the ICU, alternating with other nurses and doctors, so they have missed parts of your loved one's course. You, on the other hand, have one single focus, and may spend more time in your loved one's room than any other individual. You will be present in the room when consulting physicians come by, and likely hear their recommendations before the ICU physician. You will have a greater sense of continuity and recollection for small events and details. You will probably be the first to know when something about your family member has changed or doesn't "feel right." Often family members provide helpful insights and reminders to ICU physicians.

For example, on one occasion during multidisciplinary rounds, I made the plan to restart a patient's diet (his breathing tube had recently been removed, enabling him to eat). When we were nearing the end of the discussion with the ICU team, the patient's daughter, who had been quietly listening, reminded me that the consulting surgeon had planned a minor procedure for that afternoon, and asked whether that should prevent his eating (her father had been in the ICU long enough for her to know that often food is withheld before procedures). Had she not reminded me, his procedure and ICU discharge would likely have been delayed by a day. I was appreciative of her intervening and told her so. She was a good advocate for her father.

In some cases, it will become clear that a doctor or nurse is not competent or diligent. These cases are much more challenging and uncomfortable – but again, it is your job to be an advocate. Sometimes, if you politely and directly address the issue, you can solve it. For example, you could say to a nurse: "Tom has always had sensitive skin, and I get the feeling that it is really uncomfortable for him when you are pulling off his bandage tape. Do you have any tricks to do that more gently, or are there different types of tape that are less sticky?"

On occasion, you may need to go to someone else for help. The ICU nurse manager is a good resource, especially for nursing issues. Ask to speak with her privately and explain your concerns. Tell her who your favorite nurses are: good nurse managers try to assign nurses to patients based on their rapport with certain families. In extreme cases, you may want to request that a certain nurse not be assigned to your family member.

Concerns about physicians are harder to address, because at any one time there is usually only one on call for that specialty. In addition, physicians usually operate in a looser hierarchical structure than nurses, so it can be hard to identify a supervisor. If the ICU attending physician is of concern, you can ask the ICU nurse manager if you can speak with an "ICU medical director or section head" (this is a physician who provides general oversight to the group of ICU physicians working in the hospital). If the physician of concern is a trainee – for example, a resident or fellow – you should ask to speak with the attending physician.

If you don't get satisfaction through the avenues suggested above, ask if the hospital has a patient advocate or ombudsperson. For really egregious concerns, you could ask to speak with the Chief Nursing Officer or Chief Medical Officer – these are the hospital executives with ultimate responsibility for the quality of care delivered in the hospital. There are times when it is absolutely necessary to contact the ombudsperson or Chief Officers – but you should recognize that these are big guns. Calling on them will almost inevitably invoke the specter of a lawsuit, and change the nature of the relationship you have with the ICU staff to one that is much more self-conscious and defensive.

What can you do?

- Recognize that you not only can but also should be an advocate for your loved one. As long as you do so politely and showing respect for your caretakers' expertise and time, it will be welcomed.
- Address your questions and concerns calmly and directly to caretakers. Avoid obvious displays of skepticism – ask questions with the attitude that you are looking to learn (not to communicate doubt).
- Escalate when you have to. If you need to speak with an ICU nurse's supervisor, ask for the ICU manager. If you need to speak with an ICU physician's supervisor, ask for the Medical Director of the ICU. If you need to speak with a trainee's supervisor, ask to speak with the attending physician. If these avenues don't provide satisfaction, you may want to contact the hospital ombudsperson, Chief Nursing Officer, or Chief Medical Officer.

Becoming a "favorite family"

As discussed above, many families feel an uncomfortable tension between the need to be an advocate for their loved one, and the need to be agreeable to caretakers. But these goals are not incompatible. You can be a strong advocate while still being a "favorite family."

In addition, you can take some comfort in the fact that it really should not matter whether your physicians and nurses "like" your family. It is deeply entrenched in the culture of medicine that clinicians put the needs of their patients first, regardless of who those patients are or what they think of them. For this reason, for example, military physicians will take care of the wounded enemy just as they would their own soldiers. Daily, physicians and nurses care for violent criminals, patients whose illnesses stem directly from their own behavioral choices, and other people with whom they may not entirely sympathize. This is the medical profession's code of ethics, and it is more than just theoretical. It is very likely that your physician holds as a core belief that her professional obligations to your loved one matter more than anything personal that may transpire.

That being said, it is of course possible to either alienate or charm doctors and nurses, like any other human beings – and at the extremes of each, their behavior may be affected. What makes doctors and nurses tick? Of course, doctors and nurses are individuals, and differ widely. However, because of their intense work environment, most will be particularly appreciative if you demonstrate respect for their boundaries and time.

Medicine is a people-intense field – particularly tough on introverts. Clinicians interact with large numbers of patients and personnel daily, and many of these interactions are emotionally challenging. For doctors, it is rare to have 5 uninterrupted minutes to concentrate on any one patient: nurses, other consulting physicians, respiratory therapists, and laboratory and other staff present issues to them in rapid-fire throughout the day – through texts, pages, phone calls, emails, and in person. Often, clinicians don't even have private workspace – ICU nurses in particular are in their patients' rooms, often with visitors, throughout most of the day. It helps if families are conscious of boundaries. I recall one family member who would come to find me to ask questions when I was working in a back office, in an area meant for staff only. Although I understood his sense of pressing need, these unexpected interruptions felt like an unnecessary violation of my private space and time. Another family member managed to track down my personal email on the internet and sent me a daily barrage of messages and questions. Don't misunderstand me: my sympathies lie with families in desperate need of information – that is why I'm writing this book. But it is much better when families go through expected channels (for example, telling their nurse that they have a question for me).

Medicine is also a busy field. Although most will try not to show it, doctors and nurses are almost always in a hurry, keeping mental track of an almost endless list of shifting tasks ahead of them. The work and intensity of the day depends entirely on what patients are critically ill, and just how ill they are. Any planned activities – ICU rounds, conferences, procedures and surgeries, even meals and bathroom breaks – may be cancelled or postponed, as crises and urgent needs arise. Doctors and nurses are grateful to families who understand this, are respectful of their time, and show understanding if they are late to an appointment.

Being sensitive to the needs of your loved one's caretakers can have subtle but important effects: it may encourage them to be more present. In my experience, doctors may avoid going into certain patients' rooms – often subconsciously. Doctors are required to examine their patients physically every day, which means entering the room at least once – and certainly they also enter the room when there is an urgent reason. But there are sometimes reasons to drop by the patient's room at other, less critical times – for example, to talk to a nurse, check ventilator settings, look for something new on physical exam, or ask a question of family members. Doctors may be dissuaded from these more optional visits if they feel that they are likely to encounter a confrontational or hostile family member, or be pulled into a long conversation for which they don't have time. The best way to encourage attention for your loved one is to make it safe and pleasant for caretakers to enter. A doctor is most likely to be attentive when she believes she will be able to enter, do her work quickly, and leave after a pleasant exchange and perhaps one or two reasonably quick questions.

Obviously, you will need more time for discussion with the doctor than this. The key is to do this in a way that allows her to remain in charge of her own schedule and not feel that she is at risk of an ambush every time she passes by the room. If you have a lot of questions or need to have a complicated discussion, ask the doctor whether you could find a time to meet, at her convenience. Volunteer to be present during a certain time range (e.g., 2–5 p.m.), when she can come by as her work permits. It's all about setting expectations. Doctors recognize that you need their time, and for the most part are willing and glad to give it if they can keep some control of the timing.

What can you do?

- *Communicate with caretakers within agreed-on parameters.* Ask the nurse or doctor to identify the best general time for you to ask questions. For longer discussions, schedule a meeting ahead of time. Wait until the doctor or nurse signals that they are ready by coming to the room: don't search for them out in the common ICU/staff areas (unless of course it is an emergency). Do not contact clinicians using their personal cell phone numbers and email addresses unless specifically invited to do so.
- *Make it easy for your doctors to drop by briefly without getting "stuck."* Save long lists of questions or complicated discussions for prearranged meeting times.
- *Keep discussions with doctors efficient and to the point.* Avoid long digressions such as personal stories about the patient or your own health care experiences.
- *Be flexible and available.* Try to be sympathetic when your doctor is late for a meeting or phone call (probably, she had little control). Ask your doctor for a range of times when a conversation might be possible, rather than a specific time commitment. For example, if

she says the afternoon would be best, let her know you will be in the room from 2–5 p.m.

- *Don't overwhelm your nurse.* Avoid using the nurse call button for small needs that could wait until she is next in the room.
- *Show gratitude and respect when you feel it.* Thanks go a long way. Occasionally let caregivers know that you appreciate their care, hard work, and expertise. In particular, some families don't recognize the expertise of nurses. Avoid making nurses feel that only the doctor's opinion matters or treating them like personal assistants. Verbal thanks are much better than gifts.

Making the patient a person

I have often noted how powerful it is when family members bring in photos of my patients and hang them in the room. They remind me that this is a person – not simply a patient underneath a mass of machinery and wires, defined by the day's laboratory and physiologic data. In seconds, photos offer insights into a rich life and personality: the person fishes; he has two granddaughters; he has a giant smile that makes you want to laugh. If you are allowed to bring in photos and hang them, do so . . . they will humanize the room not only for you and your loved one but also for your ICU team.

What can you do?

- *Bring in photos of your loved one in health* – doing favorite activities, with favorite people – to hang in the room.
- *During quiet times, share your loved one's story with the nurses* – tell them about his career accomplishments, his hobbies, his character, and his quirks. You would be surprised how often these stories are shared in the nurses' break room.

INTERACTING WITH FAMILY

Some of your family members and friends may have been frequent visitors to the ICU during the first week – and now others who needed some time to make arrangements to travel may be arriving. You probably welcome the support. But you also don't have the ability right now to cope with and manage difficult family dynamics. The ICU can throw families into close proximity during an emotionally charged time when difficult decisions are necessary. This can be trouble, particularly if there is a history of discord or estrangement. On the other hand, if family members can be encouraged to put their own concerns and conflicts aside, a patient's ICU stay can be a time of shared purpose and enhanced closeness.

I have seen the ICU be the catalyst for reunions of profoundly disrupted families. On one occasion, my patient, an elderly woman, was dying from sepsis. Her son had been in jail for many years after murdering his own abusive father in order to protect his mother from domestic violence. I arranged to have him escorted from jail to be at his mother's bedside during her death. I do not know the details of what transpired between this man, his mother, and his several siblings and other relatives who were present over the course of that long night – but I do know from the tears and embraces that it was a time of closeness and forgiveness.

This is simply not the time to hash through and give vent to family discord. The more you can pull together as a family, the more useful support you can give to your loved one and the caregiver team. Families that are not getting along do not make good decisions on behalf of patients; do not communicate consistently, leading to confusion for themselves and for staff; and alienate their doctors and nurses. If there was ever a time to work together on behalf of a loved one, this is it.

If there is a history of conflict in your family, you may want to address it openly. For example: "I realize that our family has a lot of water under the bridge, and that this is a tense and difficult time for all of us. But right now, I need to ask you to put any differences aside. The most important thing now is that we all pull together to support Robert. And I need your support as well right now. When you all can't get along, it makes things much harder for me."

It is important that it is clear to everyone who the legal proxy is – whether through specific designation by the patient, or through default assignment according to the state's laws (as discussed earlier in the section "Who is going to be the medical decision-maker?" in chapter 1). Ideally, the proxy would welcome help and participation from close family members. However, depending on the family, it may be useful to set clear boundaries: at the end of the day, after all the discussion, the proxy has responsibility for the final decisions, when the patient cannot make his own.

If family members are causing extensive disruption despite your efforts, what is your recourse? The patient always has the right to limit visitors, and if the patient is unable to communicate, then the proxy assumes that right.

However, just as with other decisions made on behalf of the patient, this should be done with the patient's interest in mind (the decision-maker should not exclude a visitor based on his or her own feelings toward the person). Some states have rules that anyone who lives with the patient cannot be denied visitation.

What can you do?

- Ask your family to put tensions aside for the time being and do their best to pull together on behalf of the patient. Tell them you personally are relying on their support and positive attitude.
- Make sure the medical team and family knows who the proxy is. If another family member appears to be taking charge of decisions, pull them aside and gently remind them that although their input is important to you, the final responsibility is yours.
- Designate a single person to be primarily responsible for communication with the health care team, and have this person transmit information to the others. This makes things much more efficient and easier for everyone (including the physician and other team members), and prevents mixed messages and gaps in communication. The best person for this role is likely to be the proxy, but if the responsibility feels overwhelming he or she can assign it to someone else. Sometimes if there is a doctor or nurse in the family, that person is a good choice.
- If certain relatives are driving each other crazy, suggest "shifts" for being with the patient in the ICU that minimize their time together.

COPING MECHANISMS

Everyone has different mechanisms for coping with the strain of having a loved one in the ICU, but some coping mechanisms are very common, creating patterns in behavior and relationships between families and medical staff. Coping mechanisms are often quite functional (even essential) – but may sometimes create difficulties or misunderstandings. It may be useful to recognize your own way of coping, so you can better manage the less helpful manifestations. It may also be helpful to recognize the coping mechanisms of other family members, so that you can better understand and support them.

Frequent coping mechanisms include:

Learning

Some family members take comfort in trying to understand all the details of their loved one's condition and care. They may read books and articles, compulsively search the internet, question staff, consult experts, learn the meaning of all the data displayed on monitors (and sometimes watch them obsessively), and keep meticulous written records. This is one of the most functional coping mechanisms, and the one I myself gravitate to – I find that my heart goes out to these indefatigable, committed advocates. In some ways, I designed this book with these people most in mind. However, I would caution them that there is no way they can put themselves through all of medical school and postgraduate training in a few days. While highly functional, their particular coping mechanism puts them at risk of exhaustion. What's more, they can easily go down the wrong path, getting lost in information of questionable relevance or accuracy. And they can get so focused on details that they miss the forest for the trees. At some point, they need to trust and leave the details to their caretakers.

Avoiding

At the other extreme, some family members want little information and few details. They prefer to trust their doctors, and to relinquish the effort to understand and manage an overwhelming situation. (They may be annoyed by what they see as futile overstepping and arrogance by the "learners" described above; conversely, the learners may be irritated by what they see as hiding one's head in the sand.) These individuals are grateful for paternalism from their doctors and prefer not to be asked to make difficult decisions. While this is also a very reasonable choice, they may end up lost and confused if their physicians are not proactive with explanations. In particular, they may end up with an unrealistic understanding of the prognosis. They also will have difficulty functioning as effective advocates – it's my suspicion that these people sometimes look back on their time in the ICU with a sense of guilt about their own passivity. If you recognize that you are the kind of person who tends to want to know less rather than more, it is even more important that you have a doctor you really trust. You may want to assign another family member to serve in the role of the primary communicator with caretakers, and to keep you apprised of the situation in broad strokes.

Challenging

Some family members combat a sense of helplessness through confrontation. They take an automatic adversarial stance against the ICU team and sometimes other family members, feeling a duty to advocate constantly (even when unsure how) – sometimes by threatening litigation. My heart also goes out to these family members: they can't reconcile themselves to being out of control, which they feel as a weakness. They are terrified for their loved ones and will defend them like lionesses. In my experience, if they are given time and information by doctors and shown how they can productively contribute to decision-making and care, the antagonism evaporates. But doctors sometimes instead respond defensively, and this intensifies the problem. These family members exhaust themselves by always being in battle mode. They are less likely to hear and trust important information, and they alienate the staff. Doctors avoid entering the room when they can, and they may practice "defensive medicine" with an eye toward protecting themselves legally. That can lead to unnecessary or even dangerous tests and procedures.

Deferring

At the other extreme, some family members cope by hero-worshipping their caretakers, becoming excessively deferential and believing their doctor can do no wrong. They sometimes annoy other family members, who can't understand why they are so ingratiating and never ask the difficult questions. People who cope in this way have difficulty recognizing when they need to speak up for their loved ones.

Relying on religion

Many people in the ICU take great comfort in the idea that their loved one is in God's hands. This view is not in and of itself incompatible with being an effective advocate – but sometimes it is used as an excuse to relinquish all claim to control or need to make decisions. In particular, people may feel like they don't need to make difficult decisions about whether to use or continue life support, because in the end God will determine the outcome. Very religious people who believe in divine intervention may also have trouble acknowledging and coming to terms with the most likely course or prognosis. If religion is important to you, consider the idea that God is working through your doctors and you yourself – and that you all have an important role to play. You may want to ask your nurse if there is a chaplain or rabbi in the hospital with whom you can confer.

TIME IN THE ICU

Time in the ICU presents a paradox. On the one hand, time is essential for healing from a critical illness – indeed, much of ICU care is supportive and designed to buy time for the patient. At the same time, every day brings the risk of a new complication or setback. Being an ICU patient inherently involves risk: risk from immobility; risk from procedures; and risk from penetrating lines and tubes that bypass the body's normal mechanisms of defense against infection. Complications generally start to present themselves after several days of an ICU stay. It is not uncommon for a patient to be recovering well from an initial illness, and then suffer a major setback from a complication. Needless to say, this can be extremely discouraging and upsetting to family.

The figure shows a schematic for how I think about time in the ICU. After the initial stabilization and treatment, each patient finds his or her own intrinsic rate of improvement from the initial illness. But this trajectory is punctuated by occasional setbacks from complications. After each setback, the patient not only has to recover the lost ground – but the rate of improvement may be slower, because of weakness and deconditioning. Part of my goal as an ICU physician is to have few enough complications that the patient's underlying trajectory of improvement enables him or her finally to escape the ICU. Much of the quality of ICU care after the initial stabilization and treatment is based on paying meticulous attention to preventing complications.

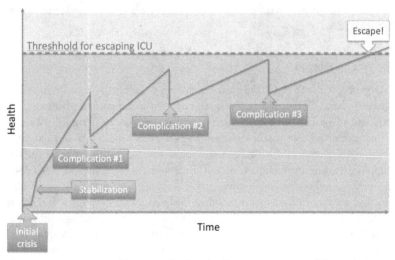

Figure 3.1.   Conceptual framework: Time in the ICU. Courtesy of the author

COMPLICATIONS

As mentioned previously, there are inherent risks to being in the ICU. For example, normally, our skin and the lining of our respiratory and GI tracts form natural barriers against the bacteria and other germs found all around us. These barriers break down with critical illness or are bypassed by lines and tubes (such as the endotracheal tube and central line), providing points of entry for germs. In addition, critical illness often reduces the body's defenses – such as immune function, blood clotting, and mobility – that normally keep us in good health. Finally, many of the medications used to treat critical illness carry risks, as do almost all procedures.

While risk is inherent to medical care – and particularly medical care in the ICU, where people are sickest and treatment is most intensive – many of these risks can be substantially reduced by taking certain measures. The administrations and boards of directors for many hospitals have adopted a "Zero-Harm" goal, to signal an institutional commitment to preventing complications. This commitment is meaningful and has likely led to decreased risk in some hospitals. However, it is important to recognize that the "zero" is aspirational. In practice, some complications are to be expected in the ICU (particularly with prolonged ICU stays), no matter how meticulous and careful your caregivers may be.

You can play a role in reducing the risk of complications, and that is the subject of this section. First, I will provide a brief description of common complications in the ICU. Then I will end the section with a summary of what I think are the most important ways you can help prevent them.

Hospital-acquired infections

These are infections that sometimes occur while in the ICU, usually because lines and tubes provide entry for germs, or because of changes in the body caused by critical illness or certain medications. Common hospital-acquired infections in the ICU are as follows:

- *Central line associated blood stream infection (CLABSI)* – Central lines and other large intravenous catheters, including hemodialysis catheters, can introduce bacteria or fungi into the bloodstream, sometimes causing sepsis. The risks of CLABSI are reduced by (1) careful sterile technique during insertion; (2) good care of the central line (such as dressing changes); and (3) removing the central line as soon as possible.

- *Catheter associated urinary tract infection (CAUTI)* – Indwelling catheters that enter the urethra and bladder can introduce bacteria or fungi into the urinary system, causing an infection and sometimes sepsis (called "urosepsis"). The risks of CAUTI are reduced by (1) careful sterile technique during insertion; (2) proper care of the tubing and collection bag, including making sure the bag stays well below the level of the patient (e.g., not placing it on the bed while moving the patient), and not breaking the sterile connections in the tubing; and (3) removing the catheter as soon as possible. Probably almost half of hospitalized patients' indwelling catheters are in place without a good medical reason;[1] they offer a great deal of convenience to both caregivers and patients. Good reasons for needing an indwelling urinary catheter in the ICU are to monitor kidney function (usually when blood pressure is low) or when an obstruction or other problem interferes with normal urination. Incontinence is not in and of itself an indication. When a urinary catheter is needed, whenever possible an "external catheter" should be used (which doesn't enter the urethra, reducing the risk of infection). These are available for both men and women.
- *Ventilator associated pneumonia (VAP)* – This complication was discussed in detail in the section "The breathing machine" in chapter 2, and will be described only briefly here. The endotracheal tube provides a direct conduit for environmental germs to enter the lower respiratory airways. Furthermore, normal defenses against respiratory infection (such as coughing and clearing mucus) are altered. In addition, certain medications commonly used in the ICU – in particular, gastric acid suppressants – may increase the risk of VAP, probably by causing an overgrowth of bacteria in the gut which can migrate into the airways. VAP can lead to serious illness and possibly sepsis.
- *Clostridioides difficile infection* – *Clostridioides difficile* (often called "*C. difficile*" or "*C. diff*") are bacteria which are commonly found in the gastrointestinal tracts of healthy people. However, certain conditions and medications can cause an overgrowth of *C. difficile*, sometimes causing a severe infection of the colon (*C. difficile* colitis). This can lead to diarrhea, abdominal pain, and severe illness, sometimes requiring surgery. Rarely, *C. difficile* is fatal. Elderly patients and those whose immune systems are suppressed are at highest risk of *C. difficile* infection. Broad spectrum or prolonged antibiotics significantly increase the risk because they inhibit the bacteria in the gut that normally compete with *C. difficile*. Gastric acid suppressants may also increase the risk of *C. difficile* infection.[2] *C. difficile* can be passed from patient to patient, usually from the hands and

clothes of visitors – so if your relative is found to have *C. difficile*, you and his caretakers will need to wear gowns and gloves while in the room.

- *Surgical site infection* – If your relative has had a surgery, there is about a 2–5 percent chance that the surgical wound can get infected.[3] Most of the preventive measures that can be taken happen just before or at the time of the surgery (for example, giving antibiotics to prevent infection).

- *Antibiotic resistance* – The antibiotics used in the ICU do treat infections, but they also promote the growth of bacteria that are resistant to those antibiotics. Highly resistant bacteria are called multi-drug resistant organisms (MDROs) and can spread from patient to patient in the ICU. Common MDROs are methicillin-resistant staphylococcus aureus (MRSA), vancomycin-resistant enterococcus (VRE), and extended spectrum beta-lactamase (ESBL) organisms. They can cause a true infection – for example, in the lungs, bloodstream, or urine – or can simply colonize the skin or the oropharynx without causing illness. Infections with MDROs are more difficult to cure than most and require long courses of very strong antibiotics. If your relative has an MDRO – whether it is colonization or true infection – anyone entering the room will be asked to wear a gown and gloves.

Gastrointestinal bleeding

Gastrointestinal (GI) bleeding can be the primary cause of an ICU admission, but it can also develop during the admission as a complication of critical illness. Critical illness can cause what is called "stress ulcers" of the lining of the gastrointestinal tract, usually in the esophagus, stomach, or upper intestine. Most stress ulcers do not cause symptoms or significant bleeding, but rarely they can be serious and require blood transfusion, or even a procedure to stop the bleeding. The risk is highest for very sick patients, for example, those who have been on mechanical ventilation for more than two days or who have problems with blood clotting. The risk of GI bleeding can be cut by more than half by using gastric acid suppressants (referred to as "GI prophylaxis"). However, there is evidence that gastric acid suppressants may increase the risk of hospital acquired infections such as VAP and *C. difficile*. For this reason, GI prophylaxis should probably be reserved for sicker ICU patients at higher risk for GI bleeding. In lower risk patients, it may be preferable to try to prevent GI bleeding with medications like sucralfate (which doesn't suppress gastric acid formation), and/or by providing liquid nutrition that protects the lining of the GI tract.

ICU delirium

Disorientation, confusion, vivid nightmares, and even hallucinations are extremely common in ICU patients. Approximately one-third of all ICU patients – and probably three-quarters of patients on mechanical ventilation – develop delirium (profound confusion and agitation) at some point during their ICU stay.[4] Understandably, this is extremely distressing to family members – and at worst, can put patients in danger (for example, if they pull out their own breathing tubes, or fall trying to get out of bed). The reasons for delirium are complex, related partly to pain and illness – but partly to the ICU environment and treatments. The ICU is inherently disorienting, filled with beeping, bright lights, and strangers coming and going. Minutes, hours, and days can seem to merge together. ICU care continues 24–7 and the patient's normal sleep cycle is usually profoundly disrupted, leading to severe sleep deprivation and fatigue. Many patients receive sedatives and pain killers that further confuse their thinking. They may be immobilized by tubes, lines, and restraints, and may not be able to speak, all of which can cause feelings of powerlessness and fear. Often, patients' contact lenses, glasses, or hearing aids are removed during the admission, but then remain forgotten in a closet. Lack of these aids leads to additional challenges in communication and understanding. ICU delirium can be prevented or minimized by (1) providing orientating conversation to remind the patient of what is happening; (2) finding ways for the person to communicate, for example, by writing on a pad, pointing to letters or words, or hand signals; (3) protecting sleep as much as possible; (4) avoiding unnecessary sedation and pain killers; (5) minimizing the use of restraints and encouraging mobility; and (6) returning glasses and hearing aids as soon as possible.

Blood clots (thromboses)

Several factors predispose ICU patients to develop blood clots. Critical illness often leads to abnormalities in the blood's clotting function. Catheters and other equipment inserted into veins and arteries provide a surface on which clots can form. In addition, immobility leads to slower flow in the veins, particularly in the legs, which predisposes to clot formation. Blood clots can cause swelling and discomfort, and at worst the swelling can even prevent adequate blood flow to that part of the body. They can also cause fever and serve as a potential site for infection.

Blood clots can also break off and migrate ("embolize") through the blood vessels to distant organs, interrupting blood flow to downstream organs. Figure 3.2 shows examples of places blood clots can form, and where they travel.

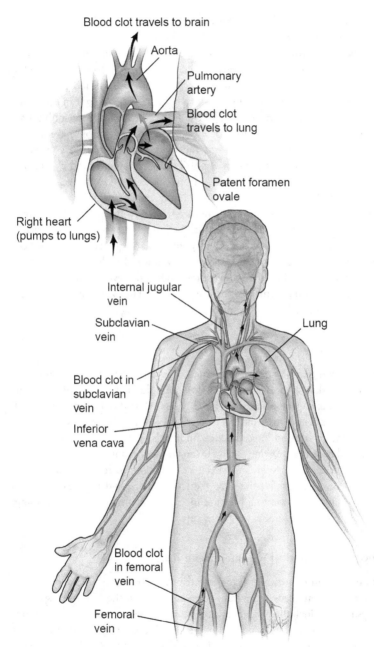

Figure 3.2. Blood clots and where they go © 2021 Laurie O'Keefe

Usually, blood clots form in the veins of the legs and pelvis and travel up through the large central vein called the inferior vena cava to the heart. Less often, they can form in the veins of the arms (usually when there is an intravenous catheter in place) and travel down to the heart. Because blood clots usually form in veins, rather than arteries, when they break loose and travel they tend to go through the right side of the heart and get caught in the vessels that send venous blood from there to the lungs. This is called a "pulmonary embolism," and it can be serious or even lethal. A few people have a small communication between the left and the right sides of the heart (a patent foramen ovale). In these people, it is possible for a venous blood clot to pass into the left, arterial side of the heart. In this case the clot can travel to organs other than the lungs – most seriously the brain, causing a stroke.

To prevent blood clots, most patients are treated from early in their admission with a low-dose blood thinner, usually administered as a daily or twice-a-day injection. Stockings that periodically inflate and squeeze the legs to keep the blood moving are often also used for prevention. In addition, as much as possible, the patient should be moved and exercised – even if that means just being moved into different positions by staff and family. Using muscles and changing position helps to prevent blood from clotting.

Pressure ulcers

Another reason that being moved frequently is important is to prevent breakdown of the skin at pressure points (for example, at the base of the spine where the skin is pressed against the mattress). For this reason, nurses will usually turn patients into a different position every two hours or so, and may provide padding around knees, ankles, and heels. Your ICU may or may not have special beds that provide some movement or rotation. Pressure ulcers can range in severity from mild, superficial skin erosion, to terrible, difficult-to-heal infections that involve the deep tissues and bone and may lead to sepsis or require surgery. Preventing pressure ulcers involves frequent repositioning, encouraging mobility, and careful skin care.

Reduced gastrointestinal (GI) movement: Ileus

Up to 60 percent of critically ill patients have impairment of movement of the GI tract, called an "ileus."[5] Several common factors in the ICU predispose to this dysmotility, including sedatives and narcotics, blood pressure medications, sepsis, neurologic injuries, swelling of the bowel, abnormal blood electrolytes and high blood glucose, lack of feeding, and immobility. An ileus can cause complications such as malnutrition, stomach acid reflux, constipation, diarrhea, abdominal pain, and an increased risk of bloodstream infection with GI bacteria. The intestine may become markedly dilated; this is called "pseudo-obstruction" (because the bowel behaves as if it were mechanically obstructed). When the dilation in the colon is massive and occurs rapidly, it is called Ogilvie's syndrome. Ogilvie's syndrome is rare but dangerous, and can cause bowel perforation, necessitating emergency surgery. GI dysmotility can be improved by correcting electrolyte and glucose abnormalities, decreasing the use of narcotics and sedatives, providing tube feeds to stimulate the bowel, encouraging patient mobility, and sometimes using medications that stimulate bowel movement.

Cholecystitis

The healthy gallbladder is active, occasionally squeezing and emptying itself of fluid into the small intestine to aid in digestion. Critical illnesses can cause the gallbladder to become relatively inert, allowing the fluid inside to become sludge; critical illness can also reduce blood flow to the gallbladder. These factors predispose to inflammation, infection, and sometimes obstruction of gallbladder drainage, even if the patient has no gallstones (called "acalculus cholecystitis" – acalculus means without stones). In severe cases, cholecystitis can lead to sepsis. Sometimes the only sign of acalculus cholecystitis is a mysterious fever arising late in the ICU admission. Occasionally, the patient develops jaundice and abdominal pain. The diagnosis is generally confirmed with ultrasound. If cholecystitis is severe, the gallbladder might have to be surgically removed, or drained with a tube that is inserted through the skin ("percutaneous drainage"). This procedure is discussed further in chapter 4.

Sinusitis

The endotracheal tube used for mechanical ventilation interferes with normal drainage from facial sinuses, and almost all patients on ventilators have fluid that accumulates in their sinuses. Occasionally, this fluid may become infected. Like cholecystitis, sinusitis is often first suspected when a mysterious fever arises late in the ICU admission, without a clear alternative source. If imaging shows fluid in the sinuses, the ICU doctor may decide to treat with antibiotics. A firm diagnosis requires using a tiny camera-guided instrument, passed deep into the nose to aspirate some of the sinus fluid. This is generally done by a specialist in ear, nose, and throat medicine (an ENT physician). The sinus fluid is sent to the lab to identify the number and type of bacteria present, and antibiotics are targeted to these bacteria.

Reactions to medications

More and more, it strikes me how cavalier we are about using medications. It is not uncommon for elderly people to take 15–20 medications. These are foreign chemicals that we are deliberately putting into our bloodstream, and we should be sure we have a good reason for taking each of them. Medical research has elucidated some of the properties and effects of drugs, but certainly not all. (Medications sold as herbal remedies and supplements are pretty much unregulated; we have very little research about the safety of these.) Many medications can cause allergic or toxic reactions, and some of them interact in complicated ways with one another. Often, medications are inadvertently dropped, added, or changed when a patient is admitted to the hospital and during subsequent transfers of care. Sometimes important medications from home are appropriately discontinued at the time of an ICU admission, but then are forgotten and not restarted, causing problems later in the hospital stay. It's small wonder that adverse drug events are the single most frequent type of complication for patients in the hospital.[6]

ICU weakness

Weakness is a very common complication of long ICU admissions – occurring in at least 1 in 4 patients who are on a ventilator for 7 or more days.[7] Partly, weakness is due to malnutrition and deconditioning. However, it is thought that critical illness itself – particularly sepsis – can cause injury to nerves and muscles. Certain medications used in the ICU, such as steroids and paralytics, may also contribute to weakness. Weakness can prolong recovery and weaning from the ventilator, and lengthen the ICU stay. It is thought that programs of early mobilization and exercise may help to prevent or reduce the degree of neuromuscular weakness. Usually, it resolves slowly, over weeks or months, or sometimes even years.

What can you do?

Preventing complications requires meticulous attention to detail, which sometimes takes a back seat to more pressing and immediate issues in the ICU. You can play a large role in helping your busy ICU team to dot all the i's and cross all the t's. Below, I have summarized the most important things you can do to reduce the risk of complications in your loved one:

- *Get lines and tubes out.* Lines and tubes – including central lines, indwelling urinary catheters, and endotracheal tubes – limit mobility and create opportunities for infection. *As soon as they are not necessary,* they should be removed. If your loved one has a central line or indwelling urinary catheter, ask your nurse and physician every day whether it can be removed. If the answer is no, ask what the reason is. (In medicalese, you could ask, "I'm curious – could you let me know the medical indication for keeping it?") Remember, many of these lines and tubes provide convenience to staff – but this is not a good reason. If your relative is on a mechanical ventilator, ask your nurse and physician each day whether your relative has had a spontaneous breathing trial (SBT) to test readiness for getting off the ventilator. If the answer is no, ask (politely) why not. (Again in medicalese, you could say: "Could you tell me what the contraindication to SBT was this morning?")
- *Help keep your loved one awake and moving.* Alertness and mobility are a patient's best friends. They help to prevent complications including blood clots, pressure ulcers, pneumonia, ileus, and weakness. Depending on your relative's condition, some degree of sedation and immobilization will be necessary (probably quite a bit for the first day or two). However, to the extent possible, sedation should be minimized and the patient should be moved or exercised. One of the logistical barriers to reducing sedation is that if your nurse has more than one patient, it may be hard for her to supervise your loved one closely enough and make sure that he is not trying to get out of bed or pulling lines and tubes. If you are able, let your nurse know that you will be able to sit with your loved one while sedation is lightened, and call her if needed.

If your relative is deeply asleep, ask your nurse whether that is because of sedatives or his underlying condition – if it is because of sedatives, ask the nurse whether it would be safe to reduce the dose. Unless there are specific reasons not to, every ICU patient who is receiving sedation should have what is called a spontaneous awakening trial (SAT) every day. In an SAT, all sedation is removed to check on the patient's underlying mental status, and to clear sedatives that may otherwise accumulate in the body. Usually SATs are conducted in the morning, often together with a test for ventilator weaning (SBT). Ask your nurse about what happened during each day's SAT.

Also ask your nurse what the daily plan for mobility is – can your relative be put in a sitting position for a while, for example, or be moved to a chair for a couple of hours? If you are strong enough, volunteer to help the nurse with turning your relative every couple of hours, or with occasional passive or active exercise. You could request that a physical therapist come teach you how to do this with your relative a couple of times a day.

- *Ensure handwashing.* Any visitors to the room, including you and caregivers, should wash their hands at the time of both entry and exit to prevent the spread of germs (including *C. difficile* and multi-drug resistant organisms). This is particularly important before touching the patient. If your caregivers or other visitors forget, gently remind them. You could do this with humor: "There is a sign in the lobby telling me to 'ask us if we've washed our hands' – well, this is me asking you!"

- *Protect sleep.* Sleep deprivation is not only miserable, but potentially harmful to health and recovery – and it is known to contribute to delirium. Ask the night shift nurse whether it would be possible to dim the lights and lower the volume of bedside alarms at night. It may also be possible to reduce the frequency of night-time inter-ruptions by staff, particularly if the patient is relatively stable. If you have the sense that your relative has stabilized and that interruptions are mostly for routine care (rather than urgent needs), ask to talk with the nurse manager. It may be possible to take measures to per-mit an extended period of uninterrupted sleep at night, for example, by reducing the frequency of checking vital signs, or by rescheduling medications, X-rays, and blood draws. (Such changes will likely need the authorization of the nurse manager.) You can also bring in an eye mask, ear plugs, a white noise machine, or music to help your relative get to sleep. Some ICUs will have a stash of eye masks and ear plugs available.

- *Assist communication and help to orient.* Good communication with your relative will help prevent ICU delirium. Talk to your rela-tive, whether or not he is clearly able to understand. Remind him frequently of what has happened, the date and time, how long he has been in the ICU, and the names of caregivers. Make sure your relative has glasses or hearing aids, if needed. If possible, put a clock, calendar, and photos within sight. If your relative is on a ventilator or is otherwise unable to speak, bring a pad of paper to see if he can write. If not, consider purchasing or creating a "communication board" with some useful words and phrases to which he can point (as discussed in the section "Communicating with your loved one" in chapter 2).

- *Give an accurate medication history.* Make sure your caregivers know about any medication allergies your loved one has, and that they have an accurate list of the names and doses of medications that he takes at home. This is particularly important at the time of admission and again during transfers between one area of the hospital to another.

- *Be on the lookout for unnecessary medications* that increase the risk of hospital acquired infections. Both gastric acid suppressants and broadspectrum antibiotics are probably greatly overused in many ICUs, and may increase the risk for infections such as *C. difficile* and pneumonia, as well as for antibiotic resistance. Gastric acid suppressants are used to reduce the risk of GI bleeding, but this is probably important only in the sickest ICU patients. Ask your caregivers whether your relative is on a gastric acid suppressant (sometimes called "GI prophylaxis"). If so, ask whether your relative requires this because of an especially high risk for GI bleeding, or whether it might be possible to use sucralfate or tube feeding instead (both of which are close to as effective in many patients). Often ICU patients require broad spectrum antibiotics when they first arrive in the ICU, but after a couple of days it may be possible to "narrow" to a more targeted antibiotic less likely to cause problems. By the second or third day of the ICU admission, it is reasonable to start asking your doctor whether antibiotic coverage has been narrowed as much as possible.

- *Question procedures.* Chapter 4 of this book discusses some of the many procedures which may be performed during an ICU stay. If you read this section, it will be clear to you that many procedures have the potential for complications. You should make sure you understand why a procedure is necessary, before giving consent. (How to have conversations about procedures and consent is discussed in detail earlier in the book, in chapter 2.) It may be useful to ask the doctor, "Would *you* want this procedure for your loved one, if you were in my situation?"

- *Use the appendix* at the end of this book, which gives a list of daily questions you can ask your caregivers to help prevent complications.

As always, you will need to feel out the right time and way to ask questions, and on some days you will probably not be able to get to all of them (which is OK . . . your ICU team will likely have these things in mind anyway). Choosing quieter times when your caregivers are not as busy will help.

4

Common Procedures for ICU Patients

This chapter of the book is meant to be used as a reference for procedures commonly performed for patients in the ICU. It should not be read in full – read only about the procedures that are relevant for your family member, and come back to this chapter of the book as needed. (Feel free to skip the chapter altogether if none of the procedures becomes relevant.)

Described procedures:

Intubation
Central venous catheter ("central line") placement
Arterial line placement
Blood transfusion
Thoracentesis and chest tube
Pulmonary artery catheterization
Bronchoscopy
Gastrointestinal endoscopy (EGD or colonoscopy)
Paracentesis
Inferior vena cava (IVC) filter
Percutaneous gallbladder drainage
Cardiac catheterization
Pacemaker placement
Intracranial pressure (ICP) monitoring
Hemodialysis

Intra-aortic balloon pump (IABP) placement
Extracorporeal membrane oxygenation (ECMO)
Tracheostomy
Long-term feeding tubes

Procedures are a common and by and large unavoidable part of intensive care. For the most part, your doctors will recommend them only when they are necessary. But almost every procedure comes with risks, and some of these are more substantial than others. Even very experienced, careful doctors can expect some complications from procedures they perform over the course of their careers. You should understand these risks when you discuss procedures with your doctors, so that you can help make good decisions on your loved one's behalf. You may want to review the second-to-last section in chapter 2, in which I discuss conversations about procedures and giving consent, and suggest a mnemonic to guide them (ROTEG: Reasons/Risks/Repeat; Options; Technique; Enthusiasm; Goals).

Below, for each procedure, I provide a description and the main risks you should be aware of and discuss with the doctor. Risks are listed according to category of frequency:

- Very common: occurs in greater than 50 percent of cases

- Common: occurs in between 10 and 50 percent of cases

- Occasional: occurs in between 2 and 10 percent of cases

- Rare: occurs in between 0.1 percent (1 in 1,000) and 2 percent of cases

- Very rare: occurs in less than 0.1 percent of cases (fewer than 1 in 1,000)

Some procedures also have a section "What can you do?" with specific recommendations.

INTUBATION

Intubation is the insertion of a breathing tube ("endotracheal tube" – often spoken as "E-T-tube") down the throat and into the large central airway called the trachea. The endotracheal tube can then be attached to a mechanical ventilator, allowing it to deliver breaths. See figure 2.1 from the section "The breathing machine" in chapter 2, to remind yourself what an endotracheal tube looks like and how it sits in the airway.

For ICU patients, the endotracheal tube is usually inserted using what is called "rapid sequence intubation." First, the patient is given oxygen to increase the level of oxygen in the blood as much as possible. Then, the patient is given a large dose of a sedative to induce unconsciousness, as well as a paralytic medication to create complete muscle relaxation in the mouth and throat – which makes intubation easier. An instrument called a laryngoscope is inserted into the mouth to push the tongue out of the way and open the airway to view. Sometimes, a video camera device is inserted to provide an even better view; this is called videolaryngoscopy. The endotracheal tube is then inserted through the vocal cords under direct visualization. The cuff near the tip of the endotracheal tube is inflated to create a soft seal against the trachea, and the endotracheal tube is hooked up to the ventilator.

The main risks are:[1]

Very common:

- Transient drop in blood pressure: This is primarily caused by sedatives and other medications used during intubation, as well as neurologic reflexes.

Occasional:

- Damage to teeth: Teeth may be chipped or dislodged by the laryngoscope.
- Superficial damage/abrasions to the soft tissues of the mouth, throat, and airway.
- Dangerously low blood pressure or cardiac arrest: This is most common in severely ill patients, especially with preexisting heart disease.

Rare:

- Severe hypertension, heart attack, or abnormal heart rhythms.
- Inhalation of stomach contents causing inflammation of the lung or pneumonia.
- Pneumothorax (collapsed lung) from high pressures in the lungs while breaths are being delivered by a bag mask.
- Severe damage to the vocal cords or soft tissues of the mouth, throat, and airway.

- Ventilator associated pneumonia: This generally occurs after several days of intubation, and may involve resistant germs that require powerful antibiotics.
- Chronic tracheal injury and narrowing (stenosis): With long-term mechanical ventilation, scar tissue or weakness of the tracheal wall may occur. This can sometimes cause obstruction of the airway, requiring surgery, placement of a tube ("stent") to hold the airway open, or a permanent tracheostomy.

Very rare:

- Jaw dislocation: This can happen when the jaw is pushed forward by the laryngoscope to open the airway to view.
- Cervical spine injury: When this happens it is usually in patients with preexisting traumatic injury to the cervical spine, or patients with spinal instability because of severe rheumatoid arthritis.
- Brain injury from low oxygen during difficult intubation.
- Erosion into the esophagus: If an endotracheal tube is in place for a long time, it can slowly erode through the wall of the trachea, creating a connection between the esophagus and the airways ("tracheoesophageal fistula"). This spills saliva, stomach secretions, and food into the lungs, causing pneumonia and lung injury. Surgery is almost always needed.

What can you do?

- If your loved one has dentures, remind the doctor, so that they can be removed (and not damaged) during the procedure.
- Say to the doctor: "I've heard that paralytics are often given during intubation. If you use a paralytic, please make sure he is completely asleep. I hate the idea of him being awake but not able to move during the procedure."
- If your loved one has severe rheumatoid arthritis or recent cervical spine injury, remind the doctor so that she can take precautions to protect the cervical spine.

CENTRAL VENOUS CATHETER ("CENTRAL LINE") PLACEMENT

A central line is a long, flexible tube or catheter, about half the diameter of a pen, that is inserted into a large vein – usually in the neck ("jugular central line"), upper chest ("subclavian central line"), or groin ("femoral central line"). Central lines were discussed briefly earlier in this book – you can refer back to figure 1.1 in chapter 1 for a reminder of the locations where central lines are typically inserted. The central line usually stays in place for a period of days, or even weeks. The main reasons for using a central line instead of a standard IV catheter are:

- Administering medications that can be irritating to smaller veins
- Measuring pressures in the large veins to monitor the patient (this provides different information than a standard "blood pressure" measurement)
- Providing access to perform hemodialysis for kidney failure, or to insert a temporary pacemaker to regulate the heart rhythm
- Obtaining blood samples without requiring repeated needle sticks

The person inserting the central line is usually a doctor, and the procedure is done at the bedside. The doctor numbs the skin with lidocaine and may give the patient some medication to make him drowsy so that he is not uncomfortable or anxious during the procedure.

The main risks are:[2]

Common:

- A blood clot forms around the catheter: These blood clots sometimes cause discomfort and swelling in the nearby limb. Rarely blood clots will break loose and travel to the lungs (pulmonary embolism) or brain (stroke), which can be serious. Blood clots are usually treated with blood thinners, sometimes for months. (For further explanation of blood clots, see the section "Complications" and figure 3.2 in chapter 3.)

Occasional:

- Damage to a nearby artery: Usually, bleeding resolves with applying pressure at the site, but can on rare occasion be severe and even require surgery.

Rare:

- A central-line associated bloodstream infection (CLABSI): The catheter introduces germs into the bloodstream, causing an infection and even sepsis.
- Pneumothorax (air around the lung): During the procedure the lining at the top of the lung (which is near the target veins) may accidentally be punctured, introducing air into the space around the lung, and causing the lung to partially collapse. To re-expand the lung, a chest tube may need to be inserted. (For further explanation of pneumothorax and chest tubes, see the section and figure 4.1 below.)

One slightly different type of central line you may hear about is called a peripherally inserted central catheter (PICC). This catheter is inserted in a smaller vessel farther down the arm, but is very long and extends into the large central veins. Although PICCs carry a similar risk of infection and perhaps a slightly higher risk of blood clots, they do not carry the same risks of lung collapse and bleeding as other central lines.

What can you do?
- Central lines are probably overused in many ICUs. Ask if a "midline" catheter could be used instead. A midline catheter is placed in a peripheral vein (rather than a large central vein), but is longer than a standard IV and usually can stay in place for many days. It has many fewer potential complications than a central line (either standard or PICC). A midline catheter may be a suitable replacement for a central line in some (but not all) ICU patients.
- *Only if your relative has chronic kidney disease and is anticipated to need long-term dialysis:* Remind the doctor to avoid PICCs and subclavian central lines if possible. These can cause damage to vessels that are important for the ability to do dialysis over the years to come.

ARTERIAL LINE PLACEMENT

An arterial catheter (or "a-line"), like a standard IV, is inserted into a vessel – but in this case the vessel is an artery rather than a vein. Arteries carry blood from the heart to the body, while veins carry blood from the body to the heart; the walls of arteries are thicker, and the pressure within them is higher. Usually an a-line is inserted into the radial artery in the wrist, but sometimes into arteries higher in the arm or in the groin. The purpose of the a-line is to monitor pressures in the artery, which essentially provides a continuous, very accurate blood pressure reading. It is also useful for measuring the concentration of certain chemicals and gases in the blood. For example, an "arterial blood gas" test provides important information about oxygen and carbon-dioxide levels in the arterial blood, which helps in the management and support of the patient's breathing. Usually, a doctor or respiratory therapist inserts the a-line in the patient's ICU room.

Risks of arterial catheters are generally small. The main risks are:[3]

Rare:

- Significant bleeding: This is usually not serious when the a-line is in the wrist or arm, but it can sometimes be serious if the a-line is in the groin.

Very rare:

- Impaired blood flow to the fingers or toes causing permanent injury or amputation.
- Infection: This occurs much less frequently than with central venous catheters.

BLOOD TRANSFUSION

Your relative may need a transfusion of blood (or components of blood, such as platelets or plasma). This is especially so if he has been admitted to the ICU because of blood loss – for example, bleeding from the stomach or intestine, or as a result of an accident – or is unable to form clots normally. Blood carries oxygen and other crucial substances to the body's vital organs – so it makes sense that maintaining an adequate blood supply is an important part of ICU care. The oxygen is carried in red blood cells, in which it is attached to a red protein called hemoglobin. In general, doctors transfuse when hemoglobin levels are less than 7–8 grams per deciliter of blood, or the hematocrit (the percentage of blood volume that consists of red blood cells) is less than 24 percent. They may transfuse at higher levels if your relative is having symptoms like shortness of breath, dizziness, or chest pain, or is bleeding rapidly.

The major risks are:[4, 5]

Occasional:

- Transfusion-related acute lung injury (TRALI): This is an immune reaction which causes inflammation in the lungs. It is usually mild and resolves over days, but it can occasionally cause respiratory failure requiring mechanical ventilation.

Rare:

- Febrile non-hemolytic transfusion reaction: This causes fever and chills, but is usually not dangerous.
- Allergic rash

Very rare:

- Hemolytic transfusion reaction: The immune system attacks the transfused blood. This occurs very rarely but is serious and can be fatal.
- Anaphylaxis: This is a severe allergic reaction.
- Infection: Transfusions can theoretically transmit infections such as hepatitis or HIV. Careful screening by blood banks now makes this extremely unlikely.

THORACENTESIS AND CHEST TUBES

The lung is like a balloon. But instead of inflating the balloon by forcing air inside, the lung is normally held in an open position – closely against the chest wall – by a vacuum seal. If air enters that tight seal, the vacuum is broken: the space between the lung and the chest wall (called the pleural space) springs open, and the lung collapses.

Air in the pleural space is called a "pneumothorax." The air can come from either inside the lung (if there is damage to the lung, for example, from pneumonia), or from outside the chest wall (if there is damage to the chest, for example, from a car crash or as a complication from a medical procedure like central line placement).

Alternatively, fluid can enter the pleural space, causing it to enlarge and compress the lung (as shown in figure 4.1). Fluid in the pleural space is called a "pleural effusion." The fluid can come from many sources – for example, bleeding, heart failure, infection (like pneumonia), or cancer.

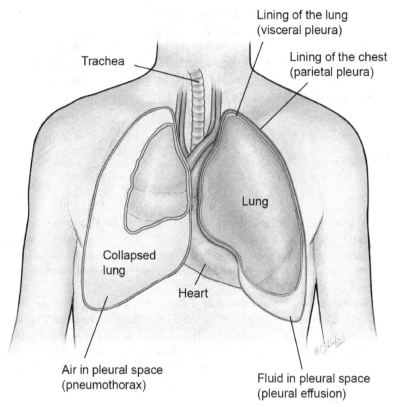

Trachea

Lining of the lung
(visceral pleura)

Lining of the chest
(parietal pleura)

Lung

Collapsed
lung

Heart

Air in pleural space
(pneumothorax)

Fluid in pleural space
(pleural effusion)

Figure 4.1. Collapsed lung and pleural fluid © 2021 Laurie O'Keefe

If there is a large volume of either air or fluid in the pleural space, it should be drained to permit re-expansion of the lung. In addition, certain types of fluid must be removed so that they don't cause either severe infection, or scarring and rigidity of the lining of the lung. If there is fluid in the pleural space, the first step is usually removing a small amount with a needle or small catheter (called a "thoracentesis"). The fluid is sent for lab analysis, which helps your doctor to figure out why the fluid is there, and how important it is that it be completely drained. Sometimes, thoracentesis alone provides sufficient drainage.

Depending on the amount of fluid and air, and the laboratory information gained from the thoracentesis, your doctors may want to drain the fluid or air with a "chest tube." This is a tube which is inserted through the ribs and into the pleural space, and which stays in place usually for several days. (Most patients have chest tubes placed routinely after surgery on the heart or lungs, in anticipation of the need to drain air and fluid.) The tube is connected to a plastic box ("atrium") that hangs under the bed. This is an ingenious device that allows the application of suction, collection of the draining pleural fluid and air, and formation of a one-way "seal" that prevents air from moving in the wrong direction back up the tube.

Thoracentesis

The main risks are:[6, 7]

Rare:

- Pneumothorax (lung collapse): The instruments used in the procedure can introduce air into the pleural space (for example, by puncturing the lung). Using ultrasound to guide the procedure reduces this risk. About one-third of the time, the pneumothorax may necessitate placement of a chest tube.
- Re-expansion pulmonary edema: Rapid re-expansion of the lung after drainage can cause inflammation and edema (fluid) in the air sacs, which behaves similarly to pneumonia. It is most often mild and resolves over a few days, but can be severe and even fatal. Although there is no firm evidence to support this practice, many physicians (including me) will limit the amount of fluid removed by thoracentesis to 1.5 liters, to reduce the risk.
- Significant bleeding from damage to blood vessels in the chest wall.

Very rare:

- Introducing a new infection into the space around the lung or the chest wall.
- Injury to nearby organs such as liver or spleen: These are severe complications, but very rare, especially when ultrasound is used to guide the procedure.

What can you do?

- Ask if the person doing the procedure will be using ultrasound
- Ask about the risk for re-expansion pulmonary edema, and whether the person doing the procedure plans to limit the amount of fluid removed

Chest tube placement

Overall, complications occur in 1–6 percent of these procedures. The main risks are:[8]

Very common:

- Discomfort and limited mobility: Chest tubes are uncomfortable and often patients require pain killers. Sedation, discomfort, and tethering by the tube all reduce mobility, which increases the risk of other complications such as blood clots and pneumonia.

Rare:

- Injury to the lung: This usually happens when chest tubes are inserted under emergency conditions. It can be serious and require surgical repair.
- Introducing a new infection into the chest wall or the space around the lung.
- Re-expansion pulmonary edema: This can occur as with thoracentesis (see description above). Generally, fluid is removed more slowly with chest tube placement, so the concern is less.

Very rare:

- Injury to nearby organs: Extremely rarely, chest tube insertion causes injury to a nearby organ such as the heart, spleen, liver, stomach, colon, or diaphragm.

What can you do?

Every day that your loved one has a chest tube in place, ask your doctor or nurse how much fluid drained over the last 24 hours, and if there is an "air leak." An air leak indicates that the injury to the lung has not yet healed. (You may want to ask your doctor to show you how to look for evidence of an air leak: bubbles in the blue fluid of the chest tube atrium.) As a generalization, if the drainage is less than 100 milliliters over 24 hours and if there is no air leak, it may be possible to remove the chest tube.

PULMONARY ARTERY CATHETERIZATION ("SWAN")

Pulmonary artery catheterization is a way to get continuous information about the heart and circulation. A very long catheter (often called a "Swan-Ganz" catheter, or "Swan" for short) is inserted under sterile technique into one of the large veins in the neck or upper chest. It is threaded first through the right side of the heart, and then out of the heart into the pulmonary artery (which takes blood from the heart into the lungs). This catheter allows measurements of pressure in the large veins, heart chambers, and the lungs' blood vessels. It can provide your doctors with useful information, for example, about the amount of intravenous fluid needed, how well the heart is working, and blood pressures in the lungs.

Although pulmonary artery catheterization provides a large amount of physiologic data, research shows that routine use does not improve survival or other outcomes – and there are significant risks, as described below. For this reason, pulmonary artery catheterization – which used to be common – is now very rarely done. It is usually reserved for circumstances in which there is a specific, important question in mind that cannot be answered otherwise.

The main risks are:[9]

Common:

- A blood clot forms around the catheter: These blood clots sometimes cause discomfort and swelling in the nearby limb. Rarely blood clots will break loose and travel to the lungs (pulmonary embolism) or brain (stroke), which can be serious. Blood clots are usually treated with blood thinners, sometimes for months. (For a reminder about blood clots, you can go back to the section "Complications" and figure 3.2, in chapter 3.)

Occasional:

- Arrhythmias: The catheter passing through the heart causes abnormal heart rhythms. Most resolve quickly on their own, but some require electrical shocks to correct the rhythm, or even full cardiac resuscitation. Special caution needs to be taken in cases in which a person has an underlying rhythm abnormality called a left bundle branch block (LBBB).

Rare:

- Infection: The catheter can introduce germs into the bloodstream, and rarely, these can affect the heart valves, requiring many weeks of antibiotic treatment.

Very rare:

- Pulmonary artery perforation: The tip of the catheter ruptures the large artery bringing blood from the heart to the lungs. This occurs only in about 3 in 10,000 people – but when it does happen, it is fatal 30–70 percent of the time.[10]
- Knotting: The catheter may loop back on itself and knot, requiring a special procedure or even a surgery for removal.
- Injury to the heart muscle, heart valve, or large vessel: These are potentially catastrophic complications, but extremely rare.

What can you do?

- Ask your physician what specific questions she has that make pulmonary artery catheterization absolutely necessary. Imprecise answers like "I just want to get more information and be able to monitor him closely" should prompt another round of questioning. For example: "Will the procedure possibly change the diagnosis, or change how you will treat him?"
- If you know that your family member has an underlying left bundle branch block (LBBB) – a specific abnormality of electrical conduction in the heart – make sure to bring that to your physician's attention. LBBB makes inserting a pulmonary artery catheter more dangerous, and requires special preparation.

BRONCHOSCOPY

Bronchoscopy is the insertion of a tube with a camera on the end into the airways (bronchi) of the lungs. In the ICU, this is often done to take samples of fluid from the lungs to send to the lab, usually to look for pneumonia. Sometimes it is done to remove thick secretions from the airways in order to improve breathing. Rarely, it is done to take a biopsy of a mass or lung tissue – to make a diagnosis of cancer, rare infections, or other lung disease.

A bronchoscopy is shown in figure 4.2.

The tube is about the diameter of a slim pen. It can be inserted through the nose or mouth (after numbing with lidocaine), or through the endotracheal tube, if the patient is on mechanical ventilation. It then passes down through the trachea, and into the small airways of the lungs. The tube has a camera on the end, which projects a video image onto a screen by the bedside. It also has small channels through which instruments can be inserted. The most common bronchoscopic procedure that is done in the ICU is a "bronchoalveolar lavage," or BAL, in which sterile fluid is squirted into a portion of the lung, and then sucked back out and sent to the lab. Lab tests can identify specific infections, and provide information about other conditions. BAL is often done in the ICU (1) when a person with pneumonia has an abnormal immune system or is not getting better as predicted, (2) when it is not clear if lung abnormalities are because of infection or another problem, or (3) to diagnose resistant infections that can occur after several days of mechanical ventilation.

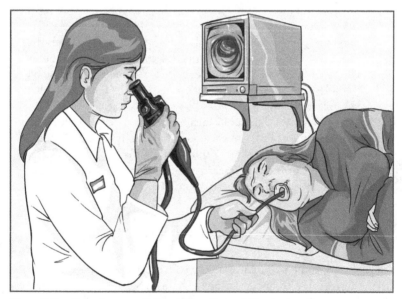

Figure 4.2.   Bronchoscopy © iStock/Getty Images Plus/corbac40

The main risks are:[11]

Common:

- Less effective breathing: The bronchoscope partially obstructs the airway, blocking full inhalation and exhalation. If oxygen levels fall, the bronchoscope can be withdrawn, usually correcting the problem – but rarely, in very sick ICU patients, this can become an emergency. If the patient was not already on a mechanical ventilator, he may need one.
- Low blood pressure: Caused by sedation for the procedure and neurologic reflexes. This is generally mild and well tolerated, but may be serious in patients who are very sick or in shock.

Occasional:
- Irritation and constriction of airways (bronchospasm): Some patients develop wheezing, cough, and labored breathing, similar to an asthma attack.

Rare:

- Pneumothorax: Rarely, the procedure damages the lung lining, allowing air to escape into the space around the lung and causing lung collapse. This almost always happens when biopsies are taken, which is rare in ICU patients. Lung collapse can be serious, but is generally treatable (with placement of a chest tube).
- Bleeding: In almost all cases, bleeding happens after biopsies, which are not typically done in ICU patients. Rarely, bleeding can be serious.

What can you do?

If the doctor recommends bronchoscopy and (1) there is no anticipation of the need for biopsy, and (2) your loved one is already on a mechanical ventilator, then the procedure is relatively safe and the patient or proxy should probably give consent. Otherwise, the risks are higher, and you may want to ask whether there are options (for example, waiting for a couple of days while giving a "best-guess" trial of treatment, to see if the patient responds).

GASTROINTESTINAL ENDOSCOPY
(EGD OR COLONOSCOPY)

A gastrointestinal (GI) endoscopy is the insertion of a tube with a camera at the end into the GI tract, either from the mouth (esophagogastroduodenoscopy, thankfully shortened to EGD or "upper endoscopy"), or from below (colonoscopy or "lower endoscopy"). GI endoscopes look very much like bronchoscopes, as shown in the figure from the previous section, but are slightly thicker (up to a little more than one centimeter wide). In the ICU, endoscopy is often done to identify a source of bleeding from the gastrointestinal tract. In some cases, it is possible to stop the bleeding using various instruments and medications passed through a channel in the endoscope (I'll refer to these as "treatment interventions"). Biopsies of abnormal tissue can also be taken. Usually, these procedures are done by a consulting physician specializing in gastroenterology, and patients are sedated. Before undergoing colonoscopy, the patient must undergo a "prep" that involves administration (by mouth or by gastric tube) of a large volume of a liquid that causes the bowel to empty stool. Conscious patients often find the volume and taste of this drink, as well as the resulting diarrhea and cramping, pretty unpleasant.

There is another specialized kind of endoscopy called endoscopic retrograde cholangiopancreatography (ERCP), done in the setting of diseases of the gallbladder or pancreas. This procedure is done less frequently than EGD or colonoscopy, and I will not discuss it here. However, if the type of endoscopy being proposed is an ERCP, you should ask your doctor to go over the risks carefully – they are higher than for other forms of endoscopy, and the degree of experience of the doctor is more important.

Overall, EGD and colonoscopy are fairly low-risk procedures. The risk of a significant complication is between 1–2 in 1,000.[12, 13] Most of the complications from colonoscopy occur in the setting of removing a growth or tumor, which is rare in the ICU setting. The risks are even lower for simple diagnostic endoscopies that do not include treatment interventions.

The main risks are:[14, 15]

Common:

- Effects of sedation: Sedation reduces blood pressure and the drive to breathe. Rarely, these effects will cause serious problems, usually in patients who are very sick, for example with preexisting lung disease or shock. Impaired breathing may rarely require mechanical ventilation (if the patient is not already on it).

Rare:

- Bleeding: This may be caused by the endoscope scraping the lining of the gastrointestinal tract, or biopsies or treatment interventions. Usually, bleeding resolves on its own, but very rarely can be serious and require another procedure or surgery.

Very rare:

- Perforation of the intestine: This usually occurs when the procedure includes biopsies or treatment interventions. It's very rare, but can be serious and even life threatening – often requiring urgent surgery.

PARACENTESIS

Normally the abdominal organs are loosely packed in fat and connective tissue, with a small amount of fluid moving freely around them. When there is an abnormally large amount of fluid, the condition is called "ascites." The most common cause of ascites is liver disease, but ascites fluid can also accumulate because of heart failure, cancer, pancreatitis, or kidney disease. Ascites fluid can become infected, which is potentially serious and can cause critical illness. This sometimes occurs in patients with cirrhosis (a type of liver disease), and is called "spontaneous bacterial peritonitis," or SBP. Rarely, so much fluid accumulates that the pressure in the abdomen leads to problems with breathing, abdominal blood flow, and organ function – this is called "abdominal compartment syndrome."

Paracentesis involves using a needle or thin catheter to withdraw ascites fluid. In the ICU, this is usually done to send the fluid to the laboratory to look for infection. Occasionally it is done to relieve pressure or symptoms related to large volumes of fluid. The procedure is usually done at the bedside by the physician, and the patient does not generally require sedation. Ultrasound may be used to identify the best site – usually the needle is inserted in the left lower abdomen, after numbing the skin. If there is a lot of ascites present, more than ten liters may be withdrawn! In these cases, the fluid is usually collected in "vacuum bottles," which are hooked to tubing connected to the needle or catheter. Ascites fluid is generally straw colored, but may be cloudy greenish or even blood tinged.

Overall, paracentesis is a low-risk procedure. The main risks are:[16]

Occasional:

- Ascites-leak: The puncture site does not heal immediately after the procedure, and ascites continue to leak out through the abdominal wall. The site usually seals itself within a few days, but it may be necessary to remove abdominal ascites with a second paracentesis to reduce the pressure and speed healing.

Rare:

- Significant drop in blood pressure: If a lot of fluid is removed, it can result in shifts of fluids out of the blood vessels. Rarely, this can cause low blood pressure, sometimes affecting kidney blood flow and function.
- Bleeding: Substantial bleeding is rare, but can occasionally be serious.
- Puncture of intestine: Because the needle is small, this is usually not a problem – but occasionally does cause infection.

Very rare:

- Infection introduced through the skin into the abdomen

INFERIOR VENA CAVA (IVC) FILTER PLACEMENT

The inferior vena cava (IVC) is the major vein that travels up through the abdomen and chest, bringing blood back to the heart from the abdomen and legs. If blood clots form in the veins of the legs or pelvis (called deep venous thromboses, or DVTs), they can break free and travel up through the IVC to the heart, and from there into the lungs (a pulmonary embolism) – or more rarely, the brain (a stroke). This can be life threatening. See figure 3.2 from chapter 3 to remind yourself of the anatomy.

Usually, if people have blood clots or are prone to form blood clots, they can be treated with blood thinners to prevent clots from forming and traveling. However, there are cases in which blood thinners don't work well, or can't be used because the patient has a particularly high risk of bleeding. Often, ICU patients will fall into these categories. For example, patients who have been severely injured in motor vehicle accidents are at particularly high risk for blood clots, but may have ongoing bleeding or a need for surgeries that make using blood thinners dangerous.

In these cases, one option is to place a small mechanical device in the IVC which acts as a filter, catching blood clots as they migrate up from the legs toward the heart and lungs. An interventional radiologist or surgeon inserts a large IV into a vein in the groin or neck, and uses a wire to push the IVC filter up into position, using X-rays or ultrasound to make sure it is in the right place. Initially these ingenious little devices are folded into a slim package – but once in place, the IVC filter springs open into position, and is secured within the IVC. Usually, the filter is a retrievable type that can be removed later or left in place as a permanent device if necessary.

Another reason for placing an IVC filter is if a patient has already had a massive clot travel to the lungs, and the doctor thinks any more clots, even small ones, would be dangerous. In this case, an IVC filter may be used as an extra precaution in addition to blood thinners.

The rate of major complications from IVC placement is low, at about 3 in 1,000 cases. The main risks are:[17]

Common:

- Blood clots: While IVC filters successfully reduce the risk of blood clots traveling to the lungs, paradoxically they increase the risk of blood clots forming in the veins of the legs and abdomen (called deep venous thromboses, or DVTs). DVTs can cause swelling and discomfort in the legs.
- Lack of retrieval: Although most patients will not need their IVC filter permanently, in practice only about one-third have their filters removed, because they are lost to follow-up or an appointment for removal is never made. Of those for whom removal is attempted, the filter is "stuck" and can't be removed in about 1 in 10 cases.[18] The success rate for filter removal drops with time, and ideally removal should be attempted within 6 weeks after placement (although an attempt can be made even years after placement).

Rare:

- Local complications at the puncture site: Bleeding, infection, or damage to the nearby vessels can occur at the puncture site in the groin or arm.
- Reaction to contrast dye: Placement of filters is often done using dye to make the veins visible on X-ray. Allergic reactions are usually mild and self-limited, but in very rare cases can be severe. Contrast dye can also cause kidney injury, especially if there are already kidney problems.

Very rare:

- Mechanical problems caused by the filter: These are dangerous complications, but thankfully occur very rarely. The filter device can perforate the wall of the IVC. The filter can also break loose and travel to the heart or lungs, or it can fracture, causing pieces to travel.

What can you do?

Assuming your family member only needs an IVC filter temporarily, the greatest risk of placement is that, with changes in caregivers, no one will remember to take it out. Making sure there is good communication and follow-up is an important thing you can do for your family member:

- Ask whether the need for an IVC filter is temporary and whether a retrievable filter will be placed.
- Ask what the reason for a filter is, and *write it down*. Three typical indications are (1) failed anticoagulation (meaning that the patient developed blood clots even while on blood thinners); (2) high risk of blood clots but unsafe to use blood thinners; (3) massive pulmonary embolism with inability to tolerate further clot burden. Having a clear understanding of the initial rationale will help future doctors make decisions about filter removal and the use of blood thinners.
- Ask what the plan for follow-up and retrieval is and *write it down*. Approximately how long will it be necessary to have the filter in place? Who will be in charge of deciding when and whether the filter should come out? Who will be in charge of scheduling the removal procedure? Remember, the chance for successful retrieval is highest in the first 6 weeks after placement.

PERCUTANEOUS GALLBLADDER DRAINAGE

Cholecystitis is inflammation of the gallbladder, and can be either the source of critical illness or a result of critical illness. People may be admitted to the ICU because of an acutely infected gallbladder and sepsis, usually in the context of gallstones. Alternatively, people with critical illness from a different source can develop gallbladder inflammation days after their admission, even without gallstones (this is called "acalculous cholecystitis," and was discussed earlier in the section "Complications" in chapter 3). It's thought that this inflammation is because of decreased movement of the gallbladder and decreased blood flow. Sometimes, the only clue is an unexplained new fever, days or weeks into the ICU stay.

Often, people in the ICU are sick enough that surgical removal of the gallbladder would be dangerous (for example, because of high bleeding risk or low blood pressure). An alternative is percutaneous drainage: placing a tube through the abdominal wall and into the gallbladder to drain the infected material. Interventional radiologists are usually the ones to do this procedure, using X-rays or ultrasound to guide them. The tube stays in place until the cholecystitis fully resolves – usually days or even weeks. If the patient has gallstones, he can be evaluated in the future (when he is healthier) for surgical removal of the gallbladder.

The main risks are:

Common:

- Blockage and dislodgement: The tube can become blocked or dislodged, sometimes requiring a second procedure.

Rare:

- Bleeding: Significant bleeding most often occurs if the patient has abnormal blood clotting or a large amount of fluid (ascites) in the abdomen.
- Sepsis: Placing the tube through infected tissue can release bacteria into the bloodstream, rarely causing a large inflammatory reaction in the body.

Very rare:

- Injury to other structures – The procedure may cause injury to the lung (causing lung collapse), to the bowel, or to the liver.

CARDIAC CATHETERIZATION

Cardiac catherization is a procedure done by a heart specialist (cardiologist), usually in the setting of a heart attack or chest pain, to look for blockages in the arteries that supply blood to the heart muscle. A catheter is threaded into an artery in the wrist or groin, and advanced under X-ray guidance into the coronary arteries that arise from the base of the aorta to supply the heart. Dye is injected into the arteries, which shows any blockages. If appropriate, a balloon can be inflated within a narrowed artery to expand it ("angioplasty"). Small mesh tubes called stents may also be placed in a coronary artery to hold it open and improve blood flow to the heart. Catheterization also allows physicians to measure the pressures in the chambers of the heart, to get a sense of how well the heart muscle and heart valves are functioning. The information collected during a catheterization can help clarify whether heart surgery (either coronary artery bypass surgery or heart valve replacement) is necessary.

After a cardiac catheterization, the catheter is removed from the artery. It is necessary to hold very firm (uncomfortably firm) pressure against the artery in the wrist or groin for at least 15 minutes and sometimes longer, which can be done either by a person pressing with her hands, or with a mechanical clamp or balloon. If the artery is in the groin, the patient will need to lie flat for several hours. An alternative to using pressure is using a special "closure device" which mechanically closes the hole created in the artery.

The risk of a major complication from a simple cardiac catheterization is actually quite low – less than 1 in 100 patients – and the risk of death is more like 1 in 1,000 patients.[19] These numbers become slightly higher if an "intervention" is done – for example, a balloon-dilation or placement of a stent. In this case, the risk of death from a complication is closer to 3 in 200 patients.[20]

The main risks are:[21]

Common:

- Bleeding: Some bleeding into the soft tissues around the access artery in the groin or arm is common. Rarely, it is severe and difficult to control, especially if it tracks into the soft tissues behind the pelvis and abdomen.

Occasional:

- Arrhythmias: The procedure can trigger abnormal heart rhythms. Most resolve quickly on their own, but some require electrical shocks to correct the rhythm, or even full cardiac resuscitation.
- Kidney problems: The dye used during the procedure can be toxic to the kidneys, and small bits of arterial plaque sometimes shower into the small vessels supplying the kidney. Significant kidney failure is much higher in patients who already have kidney dysfunction, and who have diabetes. Usually, kidney function returns to normal in about a week – but occasionally the problem persists, and rarely it requires hemodialysis.
- Coronary artery dissection: The layers of the artery wall may separate, causing a flap to partially or completely obstruct the artery; this is called a

dissection, and is particularly common after balloon angioplasty. Usually it can be treated by inserting a stent, but sometimes the flap occludes the artery and causes a heart attack.

- Heart attack: For various reasons (including coronary artery injury, spasm, or clot), the procedure may interrupt blood flow to the heart muscle, causing some damage or at worst a heart attack. A significant heart attack occurs occasionally in catheterizations involving angioplasty, stenting, or other intervention – and very rarely in simple diagnostic catheterizations.

Rare:

- Damage to the vessel used for access: The catheter used to access the artery in the groin or arm may cause an abnormal pocket bulging off the artery (aneurysm) or connection with an adjacent vein (fistula). These must sometimes be treated with another procedure or surgery.
- Stent thrombosis (clot): A stent placed in a coronary artery can become obstructed by a blood clot, blocking blood flow and causing a heart attack. For this reason, blood thinners are given during the procedure, and less powerful blood thinners (such as aspirin and/or clopidogrel) are often given for a prolonged period of time after stent placement.
- Coronary artery perforation: Rarely, angioplasty, stenting, or other interventions can rupture coronary arteries. This complication is serious and can be fatal.
- Inadequate blood flow to the limb: At the site of the arterial puncture (either in the arm or the groin), several things may happen that can impede downstream blood flow to the limb: intense vessel spasm, large clot formation, or a shower of smaller clots and plaque into the smaller vessels. If severe, these problems may require a surgery and, extremely rarely, amputation. The wrist (radial) artery is particularly prone to being blocked, but there is usually no damage because of blood flow from other arteries feeding the hand.
- Stroke: The procedure may dislodge small clots or pieces of plaque from the artery walls, which can travel (embolize) into the arteries that feed the brain, causing stroke. Tiny strokes from catheterization are common, but the large majority are asymptomatic. About 1 in 200 people will have a stroke that causes symptoms (such as weakness or speech problems).[22]
- Reaction to contrast dye: Allergic reactions are usually mild and self-limited, but in very rare cases can be severe.

Very rare:

- Damage to nearby nerves: In the groin, if there is enough bleeding, the clotted blood can compress the femoral nerve, causing numbness or weakness, which may persist for weeks or months.
- Perforation of the heart: This is an exceptionally rare complication, but obviously devastating.

What can you do?

In general, if a catheterization is recommended in the setting of the ICU, it is needed urgently, and you will probably not want to withhold consent. However, you can take the opportunity to have the following discussion:

- Let the cardiologist know if your loved one has had contrast dye before and if he has an allergy to it.
- If your loved one has problems with his kidneys, remind the cardiologist, so she can make an effort to minimize the amount of dye used.
- During the day after catheterization, help your nurse to keep an eye out for symptoms of pain and numbness in the foot or hand (downstream from the place that was used to access the artery). Watch for paleness or bluish discoloration, as well as for numbness, pain, or weakness. If you know how to check for pulses, you can do that as well.

PACEMAKER PLACEMENT

There is a focus of cells in the heart that acts as a natural pacemaker, triggering each heartbeat with a wave of electricity that travels down a network of pathways through the heart muscle. If these cells or the tissues making up these pathways become non-functional (for example, because of a heart attack or an infection), the heartbeat may become abnormal – too fast or too slow, or irregular. In worst case scenario, the abnormal heartbeat may not be adequate to pump blood effectively. In this case, your doctors may decide to insert an artificial pacemaker.

If the need for a pacemaker is urgent, the doctors may start with what's called transcutaneous pacing. Adhesive pads are placed on the chest, and the heartbeat is triggered by delivering jolts of electricity through the skin. Even with sedation, this is uncomfortable for the patient, and is done only briefly in emergencies to buy time until a longer-term solution can be found. In the ICU, the next solution is often a temporary transvenous pacer. A central line is inserted in one of the large veins of the neck, chest, or groin, and an electrical pacemaker wire is threaded through it into the heart. Some doctors will use imaging (either ultrasound or x-rays) to guide this placement. The pacemaker wire delivers pulses of electricity directly to the heart muscle, stimulating a heartbeat. It is fixed in position and remains there until it is no longer needed, or until it is replaced with a permanent pacemaker.

Overall, about 1 in 5 patients with a temporary pacemaker will have a minor or major complication. The main risks are:[23]

Occasional:

- Arrhythmia: Especially during insertion, the pacemaker wire can irritate the heart muscle and trigger an arrhythmia. Usually these are self-limited and benign, but rarely can be dangerous and even require full cardiopulmonary resuscitation.
- Disconnection or dislodgement: Not infrequently, a temporary pacemaker wire comes free of the heart wall or becomes disconnected, and abruptly stops functioning. For this reason, patients with temporary pacemakers require close monitoring.
- Infection: The intravenous catheter and pacemaker wire can introduce germs which may infect the bloodstream, heart valves, or heart muscle.
- Complications of central line placement: A large IV, usually placed in a large vein in the neck, is necessary for placement of the pacemaker. A pacemaker therefore risks all the standard complications of central lines, discussed above in the section "Central venous catheter placement."

Rare:

- Perforation of the wall of the heart: A pacemaker wire can erode through the heart muscle and exit the heart – a dangerous complication.

INTRACRANIAL PRESSURE (ICP) MONITORING

Traumatic or other types of injury to the brain (for example, stroke or brain tumor) can result in swelling or crowding that increases the pressure within the skull. This can be extremely serious, resulting in reduced blood flow to the brain and direct injury to brain structures. To some extent, doctors can reduce intracranial pressure (ICP), for example, by administering certain medications – and by adjusting the patient's position, the composition of intravenous fluids, the level of sedation, and the amount of breathing support from the ventilator. To do this optimally, however, they need to monitor the ICP.

Typically, a small catheter is surgically inserted through the skull and into one of several locations in the brain, usually one of the interior chambers of the brain (ventricles) that hold cerebral spinal fluid (CSF). This catheter is attached to a pressure transducer that continuously records ICP. In addition to the measures above, it is possible to remove small amounts of CSF through the catheter in order to decrease intracranial pressure. As a rough target, the ICP should be kept less than 22 mmHg, but this will vary among patients.

The main risks of ICP monitoring are:[24]

Common:

- Infection – Introduction of an infection into the ventricles, cerebrospinal fluid, brain, or lining of the brain occurs in up to 1 in 5 patients depending on the type of monitor.[24]

Occasional:

- Bleeding in the brain – This complication is serious and potentially catastrophic. The risk is higher for patients with blood clotting problems.

What can you do?

With some exceptions, patients with high ICP should be positioned with the head of the bed elevated. If you notice that your relative is lying flat, there is no cause for panic – but you might want to check with your nurse whether it would be better for ICP to raise the head of the bed.

HEMODIALYSIS

The kidneys perform an important role in removing just the right balance of chemicals and fluid from the body. Kidney injury is common in the ICU, and can lead to decreased urine production and accumulation of certain chemicals such as potassium, acid, and urea in the bloodstream. In addition, because of the decrease in urine released, fluid might back up into the rest of the body, causing swelling and shortness of breath. If these problems become severe, your doctors may recommend dialysis. In the ICU, the most common type of dialysis is hemodialysis, in which the patient's blood is pumped through a machine (via a large central line) to do some of the work of the kidneys. This can be done intermittently for up to several hours at a time, or continuously throughout the day. In most but not all cases, hemodialysis started during an ICU stay is needed only temporarily.

A special central line called a hemodialysis catheter is inserted into a large vein, often in the neck. This catheter has two large channels: one removes blood and sends it to the hemodialysis machine, and one returns the blood to the patient. In the hemodialysis machine, unwanted chemicals and fluids are removed, and certain chemicals may be added. Usually, a specialist in kidney disease (a nephrologist) determines the conditions of these exchanges – for example, the rate of fluid removal – before each hemodialysis session. During hemodialysis, a large machine will be by the bedside. Usually a nurse who specializes in hemodialysis will also be in the room, closely monitoring the patient and adjusting the machine settings as necessary. Usually, visitors are not permitted in the room during hemodialysis.

There are clear indications for hemodialysis, and if it is recommended it is because it is important for survival. However, it is still useful for you to understand the main risks,[25] which are:

Common:

- Imbalance of blood chemicals: Ironically, while hemodialysis is designed to correct chemical imbalances in the blood, it can sometimes cause them. Setting parameters for hemodialysis involves estimation, and sometimes a session will overshoot or undershoot – for example, for levels of phosphate, magnesium, calcium, potassium, sodium, and acid. Usually, imbalances are minor and can be corrected with electrolyte supplements or in the next hemodialysis session.
- Low blood pressure: Hemodialysis can cause blood pressures to drop. Continuous (as opposed to intermittent) hemodialysis causes smaller fluctuations, and is therefore preferred in patients with low blood pressure or with a severe head injury that requires stable blood pressures. Sometimes low blood pressure during hemodialysis requires early discontinuation of a session, or reducing the rate of fluid removal. Usually, blood pressure improves shortly after these measures.

- Hypothermia: Bringing the blood outside the body and through the machine frequently causes blood temperatures to drop. Patients may need warm blankets or external warming of blood.

Occasional:

- Complications of central line placement: A large IV, usually placed in a large vein in the neck, is necessary for hemodialysis. Hemodialysis therefore risks all the standard complications of central lines, discussed above in the section "Central venous catheter placement." These include infection. If hemodialysis is anticipated to last more than a week or two and the patient is reasonably stable, the doctor may send the patient for placement of a "tunneled catheter," usually by an interventional radiologist or surgeon. A tunneled catheter travels under the skin for a couple of inches before entering the vein, and has a lower risk of infection.

What can you do?

Ask your doctor if she anticipates needing hemodialysis for more than a week or two, and if so, whether it is possible to have a *tunneled* hemodialysis catheter to reduce infection risk.

INTRA-AORTIC BALLOON PUMP (IABP) PLACEMENT

An intra-aortic balloon is used to support patients with severe heart failure or a large heart attack, by mechanically increasing the flow of blood from the heart. A long balloon, shaped like a hotdog, is inserted into the aorta – the major artery bringing blood from the heart to the body. When the heart contracts during a beat, the balloon is abruptly collapsed, creating a suction effect that pulls more blood flow forward from the heart toward the body. When the heart is relaxed between beats, the balloon is inflated, which helps to push blood back into the arteries feeding the heart. These two phases are shown in figure 4.3.

The balloon may be used in this way with every heartbeat (1:1), or less often (for example, with every third heartbeat; 1:3). An IABP is a temporizing measure that can successfully support a patient during a heart attack or other cardiac injury, sometimes as a bridge to heart surgery. Usually, the balloon is inserted by a cardiologist through an artery in the groin, and threaded up into

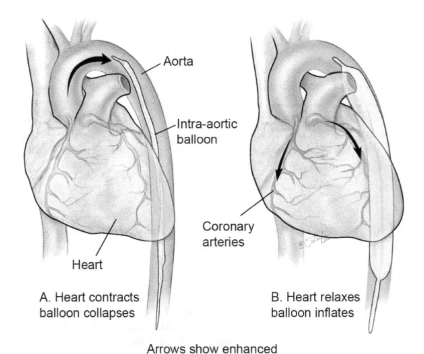

A. Heart contracts
balloon collapses

B. Heart relaxes
balloon inflates

Arrows show enhanced
blood flow

Figure 4.3.   Intra-aortic balloon pump © 2021 Laurie O'Keefe

the aorta using X-rays to guide positioning. An IABP requires the use of blood thinners to prevent clotting.

An IABP is usually used when the patient is severely ill and other options are unsatisfactory. However, it is important to understand the complications, which are not infrequent. Major complications occur in almost 3 in 100 patients, and may be life threatening.[26]

The main risks are:[27]

Common:

- Inadequate blood flow to the legs: The balloon can mechanically obstruct adequate blood flow to the legs, necessitating removal. Patients are carefully monitored and the pulses in their feet are checked frequently.

Occasional:

- Blood vessel plaque fragmentation: The action of the balloon within the aorta can cause cholesterol plaques in the vessel to break off and float downstream, blocking smaller arteries. This can damage the kidneys or cause inadequate blood flow to the feet and toes.
- Blocking blood flow to an organ: Especially if the position of the balloon shifts, it may inadvertently obstruct the takeoff of small arteries from the aorta. Rarely, this can cause extensive injury to an organ, including the kidneys, spinal cord, and brain.

Rare:

- Injury to the large vessels: Rarely, the aorta and the groin vessels may be injured, possibly causing massive bleeding.

Very rare:

- Balloon rupture: This very rare complication usually occurs because of sharp cholesterol plaque within the aorta that punctures the balloon.
- Infection: As with any foreign body in the bloodstream, there is the possibility of introducing an infection. However, the risk is much lower with structures inserted into arteries (including the aorta), compared to veins.

What can you do?

IABP requires careful monitoring, and you can help promote this by asking the right questions:

- Ask your nurse occasionally whether there has been any change in the pulses in your family member's feet. Weakening or loss of pulses suggests that the balloon is causing inadequate blood flow to the legs.
- Ask your doctor daily if the chest X-ray that day confirms good positioning of the balloon, and if the waveform on the IABP machine "looks good" (i.e., shows good coordination of balloon inflation and deflation with the heartbeat).

EXTRACORPOREAL MEMBRANE OXYGENATION (ECMO)

ECMO is an aggressive therapy used for (1) patients with severe lung disease, whose breathing cannot be adequately maintained by a mechanical ventilator; and (2) patients with severe heart disease, whose blood pressure cannot be adequately supported by medications and other means. Similar to hemodialysis, blood is removed from the patient and treated by a machine before being returned. However, instead of correcting chemical and fluid imbalances, the machine corrects the oxygen level. It also returns the blood at a high pressure, to assist blood flow. ECMO is a temporizing measure – sometimes used as a bridge to lung transplantation or heart surgery – and is generally used only for hours or a few days (although occasionally for weeks).

ECMO is used only in patients who are in acute life-threatening situations. It does carry substantial risks. The main risks are:[28]

Very common:

- Blood clots: Blood clots can form in the tubing and machinery outside the patient, and break loose and enter the patient. Patients are also more susceptible to developing clots in their own veins. Blood clots can travel to the lungs, brain, and other organs, sometimes with devastating consequences. For this reason, ECMO requires the use of blood thinners.

Common:

- Bleeding: ECMO requires the use of blood thinners. Bleeding may be serious or life threatening.
- Poor neurologic recovery: Because patients who require ECMO generally spend a prolonged period with very low oxygen levels and/or blood pressures, many do not recover full brain function. Ten percent of patients who require ECMO because of respiratory failure,[29] and as many as half of patients who require ECMO because of heart failure and severely low blood pressure,[30] will suffer some degree of brain injury.

Occasional:

- Vessel injury: When the catheters are inserted into the large artery and vein, they can rarely cause severe damage to these vessels.

TRACHEOSTOMY

If your relative is on a mechanical ventilator for a prolonged period of time, the issue of inserting a tracheostomy tube will likely be raised. As shown in figure 4.4, a tracheostomy tube enters the trachea through the neck (allowing removal of the endotracheal tube that goes through the mouth).

The advantages are several:

- Comfort and alertness: Most patients find tracheostomy much more comfortable than an endotracheal tube, and as a result it is generally possible to reduce sedation. As discussed in the section "Complications" in chapter 3, alertness helps to prevent complications.
- Quicker ventilator weaning: Breathing through a long endotracheal tube is hard work – similar to trying to breathe through a straw. Since tracheostomy tubes are shorter, they reduce the work of breathing, and may allow quicker weaning of ventilator support. Decreased sedation also contributes to faster weaning.
- Suctioning and safer ventilator discontinuation: Once the ventilator is discontinued, the tracheostomy tube allows easy suctioning of any secretions which might interfere with successful breathing. It is also easy to reconnect the ventilator quickly if necessary.
- Communication: Some patients with tracheostomies can use a special valve that allows speaking – sometimes even while still on the ventilator.
- Transfer: If they are otherwise stable, patients with tracheostomies who are on mechanical ventilators can be taken care of in non-ICU settings such as long-term ventilator-weaning facilities.

A tracheostomy is sometimes created by a surgeon in an operating room. Increasingly, however, tracheostomies are being placed by ICU doctors at the bedside, with a less invasive technique called "percutaneous tracheostomy." Almost half of patients have some kind of complication from either type of tracheostomy, but few of these cause significant harm. It is also important to recognize that the alternative is keeping the endotracheal tube, which carries its own risks.

The main risks are:[31]

Occasional:

- Significant bleeding from the tracheostomy placement site
- Infection of the tissues around the tracheostomy site

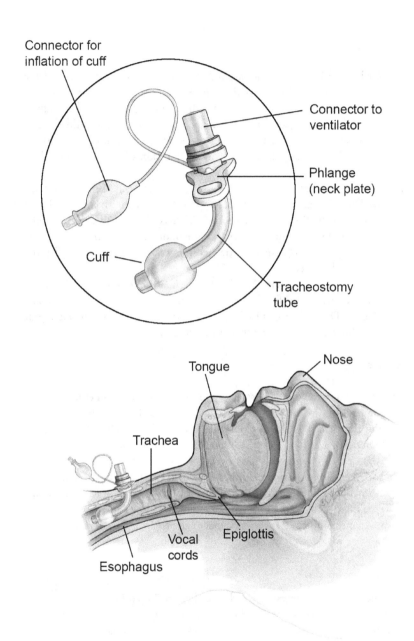

Figure 4.4. Tracheostomy © 2021 Laurie O'Keefe

Rare:

- Air leaking into the tissues around the trachea or the space around the lungs: If there is injury to the tracheal wall or mispositioning of the tracheostomy tube, air can leak into the pleural space around the lungs, causing lung collapse ("pneumothorax"). Air can also leak into the soft tissues around the heart and in the chest wall. Sometimes it is possible to feel air bubbles crackling just under the skin of the neck and chest ("crepitus").
- Chronic tracheal injury and narrowing (stenosis): With long-term mechanical ventilation, scar tissue or weakness of the tracheal wall may occur near the site of the tracheostomy. This can cause obstruction of the airway, and may require surgery, placement of a tube ("stent") to hold the airway open, or a permanent tracheostomy. Normal endotracheal tubes carry similar risks.
- Injury to a large artery: Rarely, the tracheostomy erodes into a major artery crossing the front wall of the trachea (usually the innominate artery). The resulting bleeding is catastrophic and usually fatal, but thankfully occurs in fewer than 1 in 100 patients.[32]

Very rare:

- Erosion into the esophagus: A long-term tracheostomy can erode through the wall of the trachea, creating a connection between the esophagus and the airways ("tracheoesophageal fistula"). This spills saliva, stomach secretions, and food into the lungs, causing pneumonia and lung injury. Almost always, surgery is needed to correct the defect. The risk is higher with standard endotracheal tubes than with tracheostomy tubes.
- Permanent injury to the voice: While it is very common to have trouble speaking for a couple of weeks or more after tracheostomy placement, permanent injury to the vocal cords or their nerves is very rare.

What can you do?

While there is some evidence that earlier tracheostomy (for example, after only one week) may help with ventilator weaning, there is also evidence this practice may lead to unnecessary tracheostomies in patients who might otherwise have been successfully taken off the ventilator anyway. If your doctor suggests tracheostomy before 10 days of mechanical ventilation, question her about the likelihood of your relative being weaned off the ventilator over the next week. If she thinks there is next to no chance, then it is probably reasonable to proceed with tracheostomy.

LONG-TERM FEEDING TUBES

During the ICU admission so far, your relative may well have had a short-term tube placed through the nose (nasogastric tube) or mouth (orogastric tube) that extends down into the stomach or upper intestine. For ICU patients who can't eat, these tubes are used to provide nutrition drinks and medications, as discussed in the section "Nutrition" in chapter 2.

In prolonged ICU stays, these temporary tubes are sometimes replaced with longer term gastrostomy tubes, which are inserted directly through the wall of the abdomen into the stomach by a procedure called a percutaneous gastrostomy (PG). This procedure may be done surgically in the operating room, by an interventional radiologist using under X-ray imaging, or endoscopically via a tube passed down into the stomach (called a "PEG," for percutaneous endoscopic gastrostomy) by a gastroenterology doctor or surgeon. Approximately 2–3 percent of ICU patients in the United States receive a PG.[33] Often, in patients requiring long-term mechanical ventilation, a PG is placed at the same time as a tracheostomy (often referred to as "Trach-and-PEG").

A PG is generally placed when a patient is predicted not to be able to take adequate oral nutrition for 3 weeks or more. Sometimes, the need is clear – as in cases of head and neck cancer that prevent eating, or severe and permanent problems with swallowing following a stroke or other neurologic injury. However, sometimes the need is less clear. For example, the ICU doctor may suspect that a patient will need more than 3 weeks of mechanical ventilation (preventing eating) – but as will be discussed in chapter 6, such predictions are often inaccurate. If a patient has been removed from mechanical ventilation, but testing (usually done by specialists called speech therapists) shows severe difficulty swallowing and a high risk of aspirating food contents into the lungs, a PG may be recommended. But a patient in this situation sometimes recovers swallowing function over the next week or so. In addition, swallowing tests are sometimes done with temporary feeding tubes or tracheostomies in place, and these can interfere with normal swallowing. Without all the hardware, the patient's swallowing might be just fine.

PG tubes are an example of an intervention that provides a lot of convenience to staff. It makes feeding and administering medications very simple.

In addition, if your ICU team is anticipating that your relative will need to go to a nursing, rehabilitation, or long-term care facility after discharge, having a PG in place makes it much easier to "place" the patient – some of these facilities will not accept a patient without a feeding tube. In my opinion, to prevent unnecessary delays in discharge, PGs are sometimes requested too early or for questionable indications.

What is more, PGs are not entirely benign. Depending on the medical study and definitions, complication rates are cited as between 16–70 percent.[34] The rate of serious complications is probably closer to 5 percent. In my experience, hospital staff often underestimate the risks of this common procedure.

The main risks are:[34]

Common:

- Infection: Approximately 10–30 percent of patients develop an infection around the tube site.[34, 35] In rare cases, this can be serious. Necrotizing fasciitis is a life-threatening infection that spreads rapidly along the deep layers of tissue in the abdominal wall, and requires surgery.
- Inadvertent removal: Sometimes, the tube is yanked out inadvertently – sometimes by the patient, during sleep or moments of confusion. This might simply require replacement of the tube. In some cases, however, it leads to severe infection within the abdomen and even the need for surgery.
- Leakage around the tube at the skin: Some patients will develop leakage around the tube site (called "peristomal leakage"). Not only is this messy, but it can cause severe skin irritation. Sometimes it may be necessary to remove the tube to let the tract close, and place a second tube.

Rare:

- Stomach ulcer: The end of the PG may cause injury or ulceration in the wall of the stomach.
- Stomach obstruction: If the tube migrates downward, it may block the exit from the stomach into the small intestine.

Very rare:

- Leakage around the tube within the abdomen: This can introduce stomach contents or tube feeds into the abdominal cavity, causing severe inflammation and infection – requiring antibiotics and possibly surgery.

- Significant bleeding at the PG site.
- Perforation of the esophagus or stomach during placement of the PG: These are rare complications, but serious or even fatal, usually requiring surgery.
- Injury to the colon during PG placement: This often requires surgery.

What can you do?

- Question your doctors about their degree of certainty that your relative will not be able to eat, and for how long. Generally, long-term feeding tubes are indicated when a patient can't take food by mouth for more than about 3–4 weeks. During this time and in most cases, temporary tubes through the nose or mouth can be used.
- If a feeding tube is being recommended because of problems swallowing, make sure swallowing is tested under optimal conditions – that is, when your relative is fully awake and off sedatives and painkillers; when temporary feeding tubes through the nose or mouth are removed; and when tracheostomy tubes are either removed or "downsized" to as small a tube as possible. If the swallowing trouble has occurred soon after an acute illness or injury (such as a stroke or surgery) and the patient is expected to improve, swallowing may get better rapidly. It may be worth waiting a few days.
- Ask your doctor directly whether the suggestion for a feeding tube is partly to be able to "place" your relative in a nursing or other facility after leaving the ICU. In my opinion, this is not an appropriate reason for a surgical procedure.

5

COVID-19-Specific Issues in the ICU

At the time of this writing, the COVID-19 pandemic is sweeping the globe. While COVID-19 is highly infectious and unique in its scale, many of its manifestations – acute respiratory distress syndrome (ARDS), shock, acute kidney injury – are no strangers to the ICU. In fact, ICU care for COVID-19 patients has more in common with other critical illnesses than differences. *This is true even for the mortality rate:* People think of COVID-19 as being especially deadly, but the mortality rate for COVID-19 patients with respiratory failure is probably not too far off from the mortality rate from other causes of ARDS – the unique problem is its overwhelming prevalence. Because COVID-19 shares so much with many other critical illnesses, almost all of the rest of this book is applicable to COVID-19 patients.

However, there are some unique issues that are specific to patients with COVID-19 – as well as to other ICU patients who happen to be admitted during the COVID-19 pandemic. Some of these issues are related to the virus itself, some are related to infection control and visitation policies, and some are related to stretched medical resources during the pandemic – including staff, personal protective equipment, beds, ventilators, and medications. This chapter addresses the issues unique to being in the ICU either with COVID-19, or for another reason during this challenging time.

HOW DOES THE COVID-19 VIRUS CAUSE DISEASE?

The COVID-19 virus (also called severe acute respiratory syndrome coronavirus-2, or SARS-CoV-2) is one of a family of viruses called the *Coronaviridae*, or coronaviruses. Coronaviruses are common causes of mild colds – however, three coronaviruses have mutated to become especially virulent to humans. They cause middle east respiratory syndrome (MERS), severe acute respiratory syndrome (SARS), and now coronavirus disease 2019 (COVID-19).

The COVID-19 virus binds to certain human cells that have a special protein on their surface (called ACE-2). Cells that have a lot of this protein are found in the lining of the nose, airways, lungs, and intestines, and to some extent in heart, blood vessels, and kidneys – and these cells are therefore targets for the virus. Once the virus has bound to a vulnerable cell, it enters the cell and commandeers some of the cellular content to create copies of itself. This process injures the host cell, and releases multiple copies of virus to invade adjacent cells.

The virus probably starts in the nose and upper airway in most patients, although it is possible that in some cases virus may enter through the intestine. In some patients, it then works its way down through the trachea and airways (bronchi and bronchioles), until it can invade the cells lining the tiny air sacs in the lung (alveoli). The presence of the virus and the injury to the cells of the air sacs triggers an inflammatory reaction and further injury to the lungs. Clinically, this process can progress to ARDS (discussed in the section "Common manifestations of illness in the ICU" in chapter 1), which usually requires mechanical ventilation. When autopsies have been performed on patients who had severe lung disease from COVID-19, the tissues look very much like tissues from other patients with ARDS.[1]

It isn't clear how much of the critical illness caused by COVID-19 results from actual damage to human cells by the virus, and how much is caused by the body's immune response to the virus. Initially, it was thought that the virus caused massive release of chemicals called cytokines from cells responsible for immunity. According to this theory, a "cytokine storm" is responsible for much of the damage. However, although patients with COVID-19 do often have a strong cytokine response, some evidence now suggests that it may be less strong than in other causes of sepsis and ARDS.[2] In any case, the damage to the lungs and other organs likely results from some combination of direct damage and subsequent inflammation from the immune response.

The most typical presentation of critically ill patients with COVID-19 is ARDS. But involvement of other organs is also common, including acute kidney injury, liver problems, heart problems, and abnormal blood clotting leading to problems like stroke, pulmonary embolism, or blood clots in the legs and arms. These manifestations will be discussed further in a section below.

VISITATION RESTRICTIONS DURING THE COVID-19 PANDEMIC

To me, of all the pills to swallow in our efforts to contain this pandemic, restricting visits to patients in the hospital is the most bitter.[3]

Many hospitals have imposed strict limitations on visitors, to prevent the spread of infection. This makes perfect sense: COVID-19 is prevalent in our hospitals, putting any visitor at risk – and in the other direction, it is important to protect both vulnerable hospital patients and the hospital staff who have become a precious resource. Hospitals have the potential to become "super-spreader" sites. Yet for many patients and their families, separation during hospitalization is almost unbearably painful. This is particularly true for ICU patients, who may well be in their hours of greatest need.

What does the law say? Having visitors is considered a right for patients according to federal regulations, but hospitals are given significant flexibility in placing restrictions on visitors – as long as those restrictions are clearly defined and clinically necessary to protect patients in the hospital (including for reasons of infection control).[4] Within this latitude, hospitals have created different policies based on their local situations. Most adhere roughly to guidelines created by the Centers for Medicare and Medicaid Services (CMS).[5] These state that visitors should not routinely be allowed – even to see patients *not* suspected of having COVID-19 – unless the hospital creates specific exceptions. For patients who do *not* have COVID-19, most hospitals have created such exceptions to allow visitors for patients who are actively dying, women in labor, children, and patients with disabilities. But when visitors are allowed, the duration of the visit may be restricted, usually only one visitor at a time is permitted, and sometimes the visitor must be the same person throughout the hospitalization. When patients are actively dying, many hospitals allow visitors to enter in pairs, and they may be permitted to rotate so that multiple family members can visit to say goodbye.

For patients who *do* have COVID-19 infection, visitation rules are even more restrictive. At the time of this writing, to my knowledge, no hospitals in the United States are permitting visitors to patients with COVID-19, *even when they are near death*. Instead, hospital staff members are doing their best to bring families virtually to the bedside through video conferences. Nurses and doctors, despite struggling to give medical care to increasing numbers of patients, are also providing emotional support and warm human contact. They are doing their best to take the place of families. But, of course, it is not enough. Some hospitals outside the United States are beginning to permit visitors to dying patients with COVID-19, and we may see restrictions loosen in the United States soon. I hope so. What we gain as a society in infection control might not be worth what we lose by forcing the people we love to die alone.

Strict visitation policies during the pandemic are there for a reason, and provide an important public health function. But there may be situations (in addition to active dying) in which the costs to the patient outweigh the benefits to the public. What is your recourse in the event that you feel it is especially crucial to be with your loved one – perhaps because of dementia, special caretaking needs, or some problem with communication? A legal challenge is not likely to be helpful, given the flexibility hospitals have under the law to create restrictions (the exception might be if the patient has a disability, in which case he has additional legal protections). CMS suggests that the attending physician (in your case, the ICU doctor) should be able to allow exceptions to the visitation policy, if it would provide "significant benefit to the patient's clinical care."[4] If you strongly believe that your presence is essential for unusual

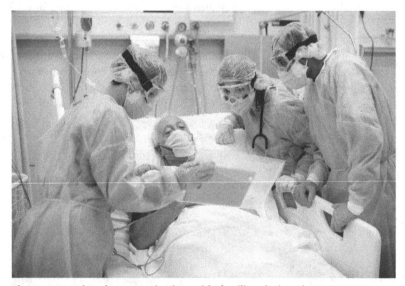

Figure 5.1. Virtual communication with families during the COVID-19 pandemic © E+/tempura

reasons, one potential recourse would be to ask your loved one's physician whether she will permit an exception. If not, you could ask to speak with the patient advocate, ombudsperson, or ethics committee representative. If you need to pull out the big guns, ask to speak with the Chief Medical Officer of the hospital. Whomever you speak to, explain why your case differs from that of the many other families with loved ones with COVID-19, and how you believe your visitation is essential to the *clinical care* of your loved one. Remember – we are all in the same boat, and exceptions will be made only for truly special circumstances.

CMS also states that hospitals should make "every effort to provide tools for virtual visits" as well as "daily virtual staff connection with a designated caregiver or family member."[4] To this end, many hospitals have purchased portable computers that can be used for video conferencing between family members and patients and staff (for example, using software programs like Zoom, Webex, Skype, or FaceTime).

This sounds daunting for some less computer-literate family members, but hospital staff can help you to set up and use the program on your computer or cell phone (once you have done it once, it is simple). You should ask about this possibility, and arrange to have a daily virtual appointment set up with the nurse. If you have difficulty getting this done, ask to speak with a patient advocate or ombudsperson. Tell them that you know CMS recommendations specify the opportunity for daily virtual communication with the medical staff. It is also reasonable to expect a daily update from the attending physician. This could be done during the video conferencing appointment, but many doctors may find it easier to call by phone when their schedules permit.

If only one person is allowed to visit, who should it be? This is the patient's decision. In some cases, however, the patient is incapacitated and cannot designate a "support person." In this case, hospital staff are supposed to accept the visitor who naturally steps into this role – and the support person does not necessarily have to be the proxy. However, in the event of a conflict between two people who want to serve this role, the proxy has the right to decide on behalf of the patient.

What can you do?

- Ask for the written policy in effect for hospital visitation during COVID-19. All hospitals are required to have one and to be able to provide the information to patients' visitors.

- If you feel there is a special reason that your visiting would provide "significant benefit to the patient's clinical care," ask the ICU doctor if she will make an exception. If she is not willing or empowered to do so, consider escalating to a patient advocate/ombudsperson or to the Chief Medical Officer. Remember that you will need to have a compelling reason that sets your situation apart from the many other families who desperately want to visit loved ones with COVID-19.
- CMS encourages hospitals to provide daily virtual visitation to patients and discussion with staff. Arrange a specific time daily to have a video conference with your loved one and his nurse. You may want to speak with a patient advocate/ombudsperson if you are having trouble scheduling virtual visitation.
- Ask your doctor directly about how best to communicate. For example, you could say: "I'm sure you understand how difficult is to not be able to visit and to be unsure what's going on. Is it reasonable to ask for you to call my cell to give me a quick update once a day? If so, I can make sure I'm available during the time period when it's most likely to work for you."

CONTACT TRACING AND QUARANTINE

If your loved one has COVID-19, it is possible that you and others in your circle will be "close contacts." This is defined by the CDC as being within 6 feet of the patient for a total of 15 minutes or more, at any time beginning 2 days before the onset of the patient's symptoms – regardless of whether a mask was worn.[6] Almost any household member should be considered a close contact; household members have a high rate of infection themselves. Hospital staff or public health department officials may question you to determine whether you meet the criteria for a close contact.

Whether or not you are identified as a close contact by others, *if you know yourself to be a close contact, you should quarantine for two weeks, and not come to the hospital (except virtually).* You should also be tested for COVID-19 – ideally between 5 and 7 days from the initial exposure, when testing results are most likely to be accurate. However, even if the test is negative, you should continue the two-week quarantine, since tests can be falsely negative (in anywhere from 5 to 40 percent of cases) – particularly in people without symptoms, early in the course of the infection. Even if you don't have symptoms and have a negative test, you can infect other patients and health care workers.

I realize that the idea of not being able to visit your loved one when they are in the ICU is excruciating. It is one of the terrible prices of this pandemic. But it is necessary and important. Another important thing you can do is to help authorities to identify other close contacts, so that they can be warned and take the appropriate steps.

Quarantine means that you stay home and keep away from others as much as is reasonably possible. Take your temperature twice a day and be on the lookout for symptoms such as fever, cough, muscle aches, diarrhea, or other cold symptoms. Call your physician if symptoms develop, so that you can be evaluated. If you do develop symptoms or test positive, you should completely separate from others (called "isolation"). This includes pets – although the rate of transmission is unclear, there have been documented COVID-19 infections of both dogs and cats, and they can potentially spread the virus. If you live with others and are isolating, you should stay in a separate room and use a separate bathroom. Do not share dishes, linens, towels, or other items. Arrange to have food delivered to you. Wash your hands frequently, and if a caretaker must enter your space, both of you should wear masks (preferably medical masks or N-95 respirators, rather than cloth) and stay at least six feet apart. Caregivers should use disposable gloves when entering your space or handling your belongings, and wash their hands immediately after removing them.

PROTECTING YOURSELF AND OTHERS WHILE VISITING THE HOSPITAL DURING THE COVID-19 PANDEMIC

One thing that is amazing to me is how much our personal behaviors really do affect the spread of COVID-19. You would think that a microscopic virus could easily find its way around those lightweight surgical masks, for example. But quite to the contrary. We have learned quickly that those hospitals that take seriously personal protective equipment (including surgical masks), hand hygiene, screening of personnel and visitors, and social distancing have *extremely low* rates of transmission of COVID-19 – while hospitals that don't have been devastated. You have your part to play in this crucial effort to make the hospital safe – and to keep yourself safe, so that you can be healthy enough to provide the support your loved one needs.

You will likely be asked to wear a mask, whether cloth or medical, at all times when you are in the hospital. You may be asked to use a designated entrance, and to stay within certain areas (primarily in the patient's room). When you enter the hospital, someone will probably take your temperature and ask you some screening questions – for example, whether you have had certain symptoms, recent travel, or exposures to anyone known to have COVID-19.

As of now, few hospitals permit visitors to patients with COVID-19 – but more and more hospitals outside the United States are doing so, and restrictions may eventually loosen in the United States. If your loved one has COVID-19 and you are permitted to visit him in the ICU, you will need to put on special personal protective equipment (PPE) before you enter the room. Putting the PPE on is called "donning"; taking the PPE off is called "doffing." There are very specific procedures for doffing, since the PPE has potentially been contaminated at that point, and you are at risk of exposure to the virus when you handle contaminated PPE.

Before you put on your PPE, if there is a window into the patient's room, give your loved one a chance to see you – wave, blow kisses, or hold up a sign. I would imagine that it may give some patients comfort to be able to see your face and familiar clothes, even if briefly and through a barrier. Your ICU may permit you to bring a laminated picture of yourself to keep in the room and pin to your gown when you are visiting. If your loved one is confused, drowsy, or disoriented, it may be difficult for him to tell people apart when they are in PPE.

The PPE you are asked to wear may vary from hospital to hospital, but in most cases it will include a respirator or medical mask, goggles or a face shield, a gown, and gloves. Respirators (such as N-95 masks) provide more protection than medical masks, but are in short supply in many hospitals; in these cases, the Centers for Disease Control and Prevention (CDC) sanctions the use of regular medical masks. Cloth masks are not adequate for visiting patients with known or suspected COVID-19, and glasses are not adequate eye protection.

In some cases, donning and doffing happens in a special room or antechamber near the patient's room. A nurse or other staff person may be there to assist you. Each hospital will have its own protocol for donning and doffing, and some will have a designated person to "train" new visitors. When you are visiting for the first time, ask if there is someone who can train you in the hospital's procedures for donning and doffing PPE.

As mentioned above, taking PPE *off* correctly – in terms of the order of steps and technique – is the most difficult and important task. Here are the steps for a doffing procedure, shown in a figure from the CDC (figure 5.2).

1. GLOVES: When you remove your gloves, the goal should be to have the skin on your hands touch only the *inside* surfaces of the gloves. Here is one way to do this: with the right hand, remove the glove on the left hand, being careful not to touch your skin. Continue to hold the

HOW TO SAFELY REMOVE PERSONAL PROTECTIVE EQUIPMENT (PPE) EXAMPLE 1

There are a variety of ways to safely remove PPE without contaminating your clothing, skin, or mucous membranes with potentially infectious materials. Here is one example. **Remove all PPE before exiting the patient room** except a respirator, if worn. Remove the respirator **after** leaving the patient room and closing the door. Remove PPE in the following sequence:

1. GLOVES

- Outside of gloves are contaminated!
- If your hands get contaminated during glove removal, immediately wash your hands or use an alcohol-based hand sanitizer
- Using a gloved hand, grasp the palm area of the other gloved hand and peel off first glove
- Hold removed glove in gloved hand
- Slide fingers of ungloved hand under remaining glove at wrist and peel off second glove over first glove
- Discard gloves in a waste container

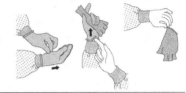

2. GOGGLES OR FACE SHIELD

- Outside of goggles or face shield are contaminated!
- If your hands get contaminated during goggle or face shield removal, immediately wash your hands or use an alcohol-based hand sanitizer
- Remove goggles or face shield from the back by lifting head band or ear pieces
- If the item is reusable, place in designated receptacle for reprocessing. Otherwise, discard in a waste container

3. GOWN

- Gown front and sleeves are contaminated!
- If your hands get contaminated during gown removal, immediately wash your hands or use an alcohol-based hand sanitizer
- Unfasten gown ties, taking care that sleeves don't contact your body when reaching for ties
- Pull gown away from neck and shoulders, touching inside of gown only
- Turn gown inside out
- Fold or roll into a bundle and discard in a waste container

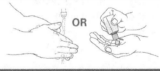

4. MASK OR RESPIRATOR

- Front of mask/respirator is contaminated — DO NOT TOUCH!
- If your hands get contaminated during mask/respirator removal, immediately wash your hands or use an alcohol-based hand sanitizer
- Grasp bottom ties or elastics of the mask/respirator, then the ones at the top, and remove without touching the front
- Discard in a waste container

5. WASH HANDS OR USE AN ALCOHOL-BASED HAND SANITIZER IMMEDIATELY AFTER REMOVING ALL PPE

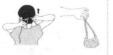 OR

PERFORM HAND HYGIENE BETWEEN STEPS IF HANDS BECOME CONTAMINATED AND IMMEDIATELY AFTER REMOVING ALL PPE

CDC

Figure 5.2. Safely removing personal protective equipment. *Source*: Centers for Disease Control and Prevention (CDC). Use of this graphic does not imply endorsement or recommendation of this publication by the CDC. Material is available on CDC website at no charge.

removed glove in the fingers of the gloved right hand. Using the non-gloved left hand, slide two fingers *under* the remaining glove at the right wrist (don't touch the outside of the glove!). Peel the right hand glove down, turning it inside out as you go, until it is inverted and covers the first glove. You can then safely grasp the inverted glove with your bare hand, and discard both gloves in a waste container.

2. GOGGLES/FACE SHIELD: The surface of your goggles or face shield should be considered at high risk for contamination. Remove the goggles or face shield, touching only the straps around your head or ears. Place the goggles or face shield in the designated receptacle (for reprocessing or for waste).

3. GOWN: The front and sleeves of your gown should be considered at high risk for contamination. The goal is to remove the gown touching only the ties and the inside, non-contaminated side of the gown. To do this, first untie the ties, and pull the gown forward and away from your body. Grasp the inside of the gown, roll it into a bundle (taking care not to touch the outside), and discard in a waste container.

4. MASK OR RESPIRATOR: The front of the mask or respirator should be considered at high risk for contamination. Grasp the bottom elastic or tie and remove. Then grasp the top elastic or tie and remove. Holding the mask by the elastic or tie, discard it in a waste container.

5. HAND HYGIENE: Before touching *anything* (especially your face!) wash your hands thoroughly with soap and water or with hand sanitizer. This is probably the most important step of all. If you are using soap and water, you should lather all surfaces of hands and wrists thoroughly, and take longer than you would think. The CDC recommends 20 seconds of handwashing (this is approximately the length of the "Happy Birthday" song, sung twice). If you are using hand sanitizer, use enough to thoroughly wet all surfaces, including between the fingers. Let the hand sanitizer air-dry (this should take at least 20 seconds) – do not rinse it off or rub it off with a towel.

What can you do?

- *Take donning and doffing procedures, hand hygiene, mask-wearing, and social distancing extremely seriously.* It may seem like an exercise in futility, but these are effective barriers between you and the infection. Otherwise, if you are spending time in the hospital, you are at risk.

- Perform hand hygiene *frequently* throughout the day . . . including when entering and exiting your relative's room, before donning PPE and after doffing PPE, before eating, and immediately after you return to your house from visits to the hospital (I take a full shower when I return from the hospital). Try to wash your hands or use hand sanitizer at least once an hour throughout the day, while in the hospital.
- If you will be visiting a patient with COVID-19, ask ICU staff if someone can train you in donning and doffing PPE and in hand hygiene, and if they have a handout summarizing these procedures. Consider bringing a large laminated picture of yourself to keep in your loved one's room, so you can pin it to your gown while you are visiting.

WHAT DO WE REALLY KNOW ABOUT COVID-19?
THE POWER OF ANECDOTES

An anecdote is a personal story. Physicians and scientists are trained to beware of "the power of the anecdote." It is a very human tendency to be convinced of something as a general truth, because it happened once to us or to someone we know and trust. So, for example, if our sister's arthritis symptoms improved after she stopped eating sugar, it is very tempting to believe that sugar causes arthritis. But her arthritis may have improved coincidentally – or maybe she just wanted to believe her arthritis was better, after working so hard to cut out sugar. What is needed to know for sure is a well-designed scientific study, with a large enough number of people enrolled to be sure the results aren't just because of chance. The power of the anecdote is legendary, and even good scientists (*especially* good scientists) work hard to resist it. All of us would do well to recognize how much power anecdotes have over our thinking, and to do our best to withhold conclusions until good scientific evidence is available.

The problem with COVID-19 is that, because it is so new, there hasn't been enough time to accumulate good evidence about it. In addition, because of the urgency, many of the normal standards for evidence have been relaxed. For example, medications and tests for COVID-19 are being used under what is called "Emergency Use Authorization" by the Food and Drug Administration (FDA). This means that the usual standards for evidence of safety and efficacy have been lowered. Similarly, scientific articles are being published online, without going through the usual rigorous process of independent review by other scientists. To the public, this is often considered a good thing; there is some feeling that scientists who insist on evidence are somehow being rigid in their ivory towers, and standing in the way of real-world progress. But it is important to recognize that in the area of medicine, actions without evidence can be dangerous. In the case of new medications, for example, you are bypassing the body's normal protections against the outside world and putting foreign substances directly into the bloodstream. Many scientists feel extremely uneasy about the corners that are being cut these days.

And in the absence of good evidence, anecdotes pour into the vacuum. The scientific and medical communities have pulled together to share information and experiences, in a storm of communication by phone, text, email, and social media. This is an extraordinary and inspirational thing – but it also means that anecdotes are being amplified and taking on more power than ever. Scientists and medical experts feel free to speculate in a way they would previously have considered embarrassing. Some physicians are changing their care from what they might usually do for patients with respiratory infections and ARDS. Anecdotes are also flying in the lay press, social media, and other public communications, leading people to try home remedies or therapies that are not supported by evidence.

At its essence and most simply, COVID-19 is a respiratory infection that causes pneumonia and ARDS. I suspect that what it has in common with the many other respiratory infections causing pneumonia and ARDS far outweighs the differences. In fact, my biggest concern about the treatment of patients with COVID-19 is not that doctors will fail to provide care adequately specific to COVID-19 – but that they will fail to provide the treatment known to be good care whether the patient has COVID-19 or not.

Here are some examples of ways in which care of patients with COVID-19 may differ from standard care – without being supported by evidence. Some of these changes reflect "the power of the anecdote"; others reflect understandable concern about preventing the spread of infection in the hospital.

Changing the timing of mechanical ventilation

Early in the COVID-19 pandemic, it was suggested that patients with COVID-19 pneumonia should be started on mechanical ventilation sooner than other patients would be. The argument was that once respiratory deterioration began, mechanical ventilation was nearly inevitable, and earlier intubation would reduce the risk of contagion. Now, a contrary school of thought holds that patients with COVID-19 "don't do well" on ventilators, and it is better to try to avoid mechanical ventilation as long as possible. There is no good evidence to support either idea. As with other patients, it is almost certainly better to start mechanical ventilation early enough to avoid a last-minute scramble and exhausting the patient with the struggle to breathe – but late enough to give the patient a chance to avoid mechanical ventilation altogether. In addition to changes in the timing of mechanical ventilation, there are shifting standards for whether mechanical ventilation should be started at all. I talk about this more in a later section of this chapter.

Treating ARDS differently

Anecdotes and some small studies suggest that the lungs of COVID-19 patients may not be as stiff as the lungs of other patients with ARDS. Other anecdotes suggest that, consistent with this lack of stiffness, patients respond better to higher pressures delivered by the ventilator. Still other anecdotes suggest that patients respond well to early "proning" – that is, turning the patient on his or her stomach, which redistributes fluid and blood flow in the lungs. Proning has long been shown to improve oxygen levels in the blood for patients with ARDS, but studies have so far not conclusively shown a benefit in terms of survival. (One much-quoted large clinical trial showed a survival benefit, but this result has been questioned.[7]) Proning is also associated with many dangers to the patient, such as inadvertent dislodgement of the breathing tube. Yet, despite the lack of strong evidence and the risks, many hospitals have implemented protocols for early proning of patients with COVID-19. In my opinion, both higher ventilator pressures and proning should probably be used as they have always been in the past – based on the physiology and response of the individual patient, not based on the cause of their ARDS. As more data accumulates, there is increasing recognition that, in fact, ARDS caused by COVID-19 behaves very similarly to ARDS caused by other conditions.[8, 9, 10]

Treating the body's inflammatory response differently

Many have hypothesized that an important cause of critical illness in COVID-19 is an overly exuberant inflammatory response, in which the body's immune system releases a huge amount of cytokines (in a "cytokine storm"). For this reason, some doctors started treating patients with COVID-19 with immune suppressant medications that target specific cytokines, such as inhibitors of the cytokine interleukin-6 (IL-6). Subsequently, these medications were shown to be ineffective (although steroids, which are more general immune suppressants, may be helpful, as I'll discuss later). In addition, some studies have now shown that the cytokine release with COVID-19 is actually less than that in sepsis or other causes of ARDS.[2]

Giving higher doses of blood thinners to prevent blood clots

Good evidence suggests that COVID-19 predisposes patients to getting blood clots that can cause serious problems like pulmonary embolism (clots in the lung blood vessels) and stroke. For this reason, some physicians treat patients with higher than usual doses of blood thinners, to prevent such clots. The problem with this is that blood thinners are themselves risky, because they can cause serious bleeding complications. We don't yet have enough evidence to know whether treating with higher-dose blood thinners to prevent clots causes more good than harm. In fact, some early evidence has now reportedly shown that higher dose blood thinners may cause more harm than good in critically ill patients with COVID-19.[11]

Using more sedation

Doctors and nurses are sharing stories that critically ill patients with COVID-19 require higher than usual doses of sedatives to achieve the same level of sedation. In addition, some are advocating targeting a deeper level of sedation than for other patients with ARDS (in part to reduce the risk of patients pulling their endotracheal tubes out, which risks exposing medical staff to infection). This is despite the fact that we *do* know that deeper sedation is associated with more ICU delirium, longer ICU stays, and possibly even higher mortality. Under normal circumstances, minimizing sedation as much as possible is part of basic, good ICU care.

Changing cardiopulmonary resuscitation methods

As the science of cardiopulmonary resuscitation has progressed, it has become clear that immediate chest compressions and cardiac support should be prioritized over supporting the patient's breathing. Now, under standard CPR protocols, patients usually don't receive support for breathing until 30 seconds after the "code" begins. Usually in the hospital, breaths are initially delivered using a device called a bag mask – but this creates the risk of aerosolizing COVID-19 virus and infecting people in the room. Some hospitals have gone so far as to suggest that patients with COVID-19 who are not breathing should not receive *any* supported breaths until a breathing tube can be inserted and a ventilator attached (which is a closed circuit, and less risky for bystanders). While it is true that patients can wait a lot longer for breaths to be delivered than we once thought, in many cases it may not be possible to wait to insert a breathing tube.

Reducing hands-on care

This category of change doesn't reflect the power of the anecdote; rather it reflects understandable concern about infection control. Caregivers seek to minimize in-person contact with patients with COVID-19. This is entirely reasonable, given the contagion risks, the shortages of masks and other PPE, and the rituals associated with going into and out of the room. But it may affect things that are important to the patient. For example, physicians and nurses may examine patients less frequently, making them less likely to notice important findings or complications. Mobilizing patients – including turning them, moving arms and legs, moving them to a sitting position or out of bed to a chair, or having them stand or even walk – has become a standard part of regular ICU care, because it may reduce complications and shorten length of stay. But caretakers may be less likely to do this in the setting of COVID-19. Physicians may preferentially prescribe drugs or treatments that are given infrequently. ICU teams may be more likely to prefer a feeding tube, rather than to provide the bedside care necessary for oral feeding. Nurses and respiratory therapists may be less likely to check on alarms and equipment – or do bandage changes, mouth care, hygiene, or other non-urgent kinds of care that have important functions. All caretakers may be less likely to provide the personal contact and communication needed for comforting and orienting the patient.

What can you do?

Recognize the pull that "anecdotes" will have on you, especially right now when you are desperate for something to help your loved one. Try to resist the influence of the many stories flying by word of mouth and on the internet, and instead rely on your doctor's best assessment of available evidence. But don't be shy about asking her whether there is strong evidence for something she suggests. Medications and treatments that have not been rigorously proven to be effective and safe *may be neither*.

THE LITTLE WE *DO* KNOW –
COVID-19-SPECIFIC THERAPIES

The most important thing we can do for critically ill patients with COVID-19 is the most important thing we do for all patients: provide thorough, meticulous, evidence-based ICU care to support patients until their bodies can overcome the infection. In particular, we should ensure we do the evidence-based things we have always done to manage ARDS, most importantly delivering low volume breaths from the ventilator ("low tidal volume ventilation") to avoid stretching and further injuring the lung. (See the section "Common manifestations of illness in the ICU" in chapter 1 to review ARDS.) In general, we should be doing our best not to deviate from our usual standards of care. But in addition, enough evidence is finally accumulating to support a few COVID-19-specific therapies.

At the time of this writing, the therapy most conclusively shown to improve survival for patients with COVID-19 is steroid treatment. Most of the evidence is from a single large study, so as more studies are done, this may change. But at this point it appears that treating with steroids reduces mortality in COVID-19 patients with pneumonia by about 17 percent. (The benefit seems to be primarily for patients with severe pneumonia, requiring oxygen treatment – other patients may actually do worse with steroids.[12]) There is also some early evidence that other drugs that target the immune response to COVID-19 (such as inhibitors of the cytokine interleukin-6) may provide added benefit when used in combination with steroids.[12]

Another therapy that has been shown to confer some benefit is an antiviral medication called remdesivir. In patients who are early in their course or are on only small amounts of oxygen, it appears that treating with remdesivir can cut recovery time by about a third.[13] There is as of yet no clear evidence of a survival benefit.[14]

In addition, we do have some accumulating evidence suggesting that therapies that initially seemed hopeful actually are *not* effective – and in some cases cause harm. These therapies include hydroxychloroquine, azithromycin, and the antiviral lopinavir-ritonavir.

This field is advancing rapidly, and by the time this book is in print we will certainly know more. Therapies that involve giving antibodies against COVID-19 (for example, by transfusing the plasma of someone who has recovered from COVID-19, called "convalescent plasma") seem promising, but have not yet been proven effective. Clinical trials of these and many more therapies are ongoing.

People often assume that enrolling in a clinical trial will give them a personal advantage as a patient – and it is true that a clinical trial often comes with more attention and closer follow-up from doctors and researchers. However, it is also true that most new therapies tested in clinical trials end up being found *not* to be better than the gold standard against which they are tested[15, 16] – and sometimes they are even found to be harmful. It seems counterintuitive, but participating in a trial may actually worsen your chances compared to the current best treatment. In addition, being in a trial limits your flexibility to start or stop treatments, based on your individual circumstances.

In general, therefore, I think patients should be cautious about enrolling in trials. However, if there was ever a time to consider enrolling in a trial, that time is now. To be clear, this is for the sake of public health, not for personal benefit. The need for better knowledge about this devastating virus is pressing. If you or your family member has COVID-19, enrolling in one of the many existing clinical trials is something important that you can do for humankind. Particularly if your doctor suggests using one of the non-proven treatments, ask whether this could be done through a clinical trial.

What can you do?

- Recognize that the most important part of your loved one's care is standard supportive care.
- At the time of this writing, there are few therapies specific to COVID-19 that have been shown to be of benefit. These include steroids (possibly together with another immune modifier) and remdesivir. Information will likely change rapidly.
- At the time of this writing, the most effective treatment appears to be steroids. If your loved one is on oxygen or mechanical ventilation, ask the doctor if steroids have been started.
- Let your physician know if you think your loved one would be willing to be entered in a research study. Current federally funded clinical trials are listed on the NIH website ClinicalTrials.gov.

COVID-19 CRITICAL ILLNESS

Most patients with COVID-19 who become critically ill have ARDS. ARDS is reviewed in the section "Common manifestations of illness in the ICU" in chapter 1. It is an inflammatory injury to the lungs which can be triggered by multiple conditions, including major trauma (such as from a car crash), severe infections anywhere in the body, and certain toxins and drugs. Severe respiratory infections, including viral infections like flu, can cause ARDS.

The problem that brings most COVID-19 patients to the ICU is difficulty breathing. Before ICU admission, these patients may actually have started to feel better after their initial symptoms (for example, fever, cough, and fatigue), but start to become short of breath about a week later. Shortness of breath can progress rapidly and become full-blown ARDS over the next 2–3 days. As with ARDS from other causes, patients with COVID-19-induced ARDS have a slow course. The median time that these patients are on a mechanical ventilator is 2 weeks,[7] and sometimes mechanical ventilation is required for more than a month. If your loved one has been admitted with ARDS, you will need to be prepared for the possibility of a long haul.

Most ICU care will revolve around supporting your loved one while his lungs slowly heal, and trying to prevent the complications that are frequent with long ICU stays (as described in chapter 3). There are some complications that are unique or particularly prominent in COVID-19 critical illness. For many of these, it is not clear whether they are the result of direct effects of the virus on the body, or indirect effects of critical illness and the body's inflammatory response.

Heart problems occur in about a quarter of COVID-19 patients in the ICU. Often, they develop only after a week or two after ICU admission, after ARDS has already started to improve. This can be an agonizing setback for family members, who may have just begun to feel optimistic about a full recovery. Heart problems can range from fairly benign arrhythmias (irregular heartbeats), to heart attacks, to disease of the heart muscle ("cardiomyopathy") with resultant heart failure, shock, and even cardiac arrest.

Acute kidney injury is also common, occurring in about a third of ICU patients with COVID-19, and almost universally in those who are on mechanical ventilation. Usually, kidney problems begin within a day of arrival in the ICU. Many of these patients will require hemodialysis (see "Common manifestations of illness in the ICU" in chapter 1 for a discussion of acute kidney injury, and chapter 4 for a discussion of hemodialysis).

It is also common to develop mental problems, such as severe agitation and confusion. This will, of course, be distressing to you. Many critically ill patients with COVID-19 require high doses of sedatives to feel calm and be safe. Remember that delirium is also common in other severe illness. It is not clear yet whether delirium in COVID-19 represents a direct effect of the virus, or the normal physiologic response to critical illness, medications, and the ICU environment.

Blood clots are also common complications in the ICU (as described in chapter 3), and appear to happen especially frequently in ICU patients with COVID-19 – in as many as one-third of them.[17] Often, these clots are found in large vessels of the legs and arms, sometimes associated with an intravenous catheter. Occasionally, clots may travel to important organs like the lungs ("pulmonary embolism") or brain ("stroke"). To prevent clots, your relative's doctor will probably prescribe small doses of a blood thinner every day.

PROGNOSIS FOR PATIENTS CRITICALLY ILL WITH COVID-19

It is difficult to estimate the mortality rate for COVID-19 infection, since many infected people don't have symptoms and are therefore not counted. However, including asymptomatic people, the overall mortality rate is probably less than 1 percent.[18] Among patients who are sick enough from COVID-19 to be admitted to an ICU, reported mortality rates vary widely – from 12 percent to 78 percent![19] This likely reflects the highly variable settings and conditions of ICUs across the world during the pandemic, as well as improvements in managing the disease over time. One large study that is probably representative of many urban U.S. hospitals suggested a hospital mortality rate of 23 percent for all ICU patients with COVID-19.[20] Another recent study in the United States found that among COVID-19 patients put on mechanical ventilation (almost always for ARDS), the hospital mortality rate is 36 percent.[21]

While this is certainly sobering, it is important to put these mortality rates in perspective by comparing them to mortality for ICU patients in general. Average mortality for all ICU patients in the Unites States ranges from about 10 to 20 percent – not too far off from 23 percent. And mortality from ARDS (from causes other than COVID-19) is usually reported in the range of 30–40 percent – consistent with the 36 percent found in the study of COVID-19 patients mentioned above. The ICU is *meant* for very sick people. COVID-19 is serious, but not a death sentence: it is worth the same kind of aggressive care that we use for other serious conditions. (The real question is, do we have the resources to provide that level of care for so many patients at once?)

The risk of death from COVID-19 increases steeply with age. It is also higher for patients with other comorbidities such as obesity, heart disease, diabetes, hypertension, lung diseases, cancer, and chronic kidney failure. This is also true for patients with ARDS from other causes (although it appears the effect of age may be particularly pronounced for COVID-19). African American/Black and Hispanic populations are more likely to contract COVID-19, probably because they are more likely to be exposed to the virus, but once they have it, they have similar mortality rates.[22]

Many ICU patients with COVID-19 can expect a long course in the ICU, particularly if they have ARDS and require mechanical ventilation. About half of these patients require a ventilator for more than 2 weeks – and some may be on the ventilator for several weeks or even months.[23] Many patients are eventually discharged to inpatient rehabilitation units, or to long-term acute care facilities – including specialized facilities for weaning patients off mechanical ventilation.

For most COVID-19 patients, the typical time to recovery is 3–6 weeks – but many still have some symptoms, such as dyspnea, fatigue, joint pains, chest pain, and memory and sleep problems, several months after the onset of their illness. What about the sickest COVID-19 patients, who were in the ICU? What can they expect after discharge? At the time of this writing, we are just beginning to get some long-term information – and it is also probably valid to extrapolate from what we know from patients with ARDS from other causes.

Patients with ARDS from any cause often have persistent aftereffects from their critical illness. These include a high rate of what is called the post-intensive care syndrome, or "PICS," in which patients have persistent problems in aspects of cognition, mental health, or physical function. (PICS is discussed in more detail in chapter 8.) More than one-third of ARDS patients have persistent problems with thinking and understanding – for example, with memory, concentration, managing logistics and finances, reading, and following conversations.[24] These impairments tend to improve somewhat over the first year, but can persist for years. More than a third of patients with ARDS have persistent psychiatric problems including depression, insomnia, and post-traumatic stress disorder, and almost two-thirds have persistent anxiety.[25] Some predict that COVID-19 patients may have additional psychiatric effects, because of the special issues of isolation from family and caregivers, and perceived stigmatization. From the largest study of follow-up symptoms that we have at the time of this writing, it appears that about a third of patients with severe COVID-19 have persistent anxiety or depression six months after discharge.[26] (This is fairly consistent with the data about ARDS from other causes.)

Finally, many ARDS patients develop physical problems such muscle weakness or contractures (tightening of tissues around joints) that interfere with activities. These problems usually improve over a couple of years after the hospitalization, but often don't fully resolve. Two years after an ICU admission for ARDS, for example, patients walk at a slower pace than average for healthy people of the same age and sex,[27] and about two-thirds of them require assistance for at least two important activities of daily living (cooking, cleaning, transportation, laundry, and managing finances).[28] Such issues may be exacerbated for patients with ARDS from COVID-19, because these patients tend to be on mechanical ventilation for a long time, and may receive more therapies that are associated with ICU-acquired weakness (like heavy sedation and steroids). The largest follow-up study to date shows that after six months, the large majority (81 percent) of patients who were severely ill with COVID-19 still have fatigue or weakness, and 29 percent walk more slowly than predicted on testing.[21]

ARDS patients may also have persistent problems with shortness of breath and exercise tolerance after discharge, because of the injury to their lungs, and they may require supplemental oxygen for some time. Consistent with this, it has been shown that six months after discharge, more than half of severely ill COVID-19 patients have evidence on testing of impaired lung function.[21] Generally, lung function improves steadily after ARDS, with complete normalization in most patients by five years after hospitalization.[21] But a few patients never return completely to baseline.

STRAINED RESOURCES

As discussed earlier, much of the clinical problems and ICU care for patients with COVID-19 is similar to that for other critical illnesses causing ARDS. What makes this illness so different from others is not so much its effect on the functioning of the body, but its effect on the functioning of our health care system – because so many patients are flooding our hospitals at once.

Hospitals have been forced to take measures to expand their capacity rapidly. They have created makeshift ICUs in places like emergency rooms and operating rooms, which aren't necessarily ideally equipped for long-term care of the critically ill. They have had to staff ICUs with nurses and physicians who have no specialty training and little experience in ICU care. Nurses and physicians are caring for many more patients than they are accustomed to, and working more hours. When mechanical ventilators start to be in short supply, hospitals convert anesthesia machines or machines used for sleep apnea into simple ventilators. In some cases, ICUs have had to use mechanical ventilators for more than one patient at a time. This is possible, but complicated and problematic, because unless the two patients happen to be closely matched in terms of their lung function, the volume and pressure of delivered breaths will be ideal for neither.

In short, it is a reality during this pandemic that critically ill patients are receiving care in a situation of understaffing, mismatched expertise, inadequate equipment, and on-the-fly troubleshooting. This will undoubtedly affect your experience in the ICU, regardless of whether your loved one has COVID-19 infection. It is important to remember that your doctors and nurses are doing the very best they can under tremendously difficult circumstances. They will have no choice but to cut corners – and one of the first corners they will cut is probably the quality of communication with the families of their patients. Be patient with them, and realize that they are trying to make room for the most pressing aspects of patients' care.

RATIONING

Most disturbingly, despite all the measures to expand capacity, some hospitals across the world have found themselves forced to ration ventilators and ICU beds. Initially, these terrible decisions took the world by surprise, and fell to individual doctors to make on a case-by-case basis. This was morally unacceptable and traumatic to many physicians. Many health care organizations have now developed protocols for rationing to try to make the process fairer and more objective, and to take the responsibility off individual doctors. Such protocols are implemented when resources are maximally strained, and they prioritize patients based on severity of illness and likelihood of surviving with the help of life support (using criteria such as severity of illness, age, etc.). They may address decisions both about who is put on a ventilator in the first place, and when ventilator support is withdrawn when a patient isn't getting better.

But even before such rationing protocols are officially triggered, "soft" rationing probably starts to happen. Physicians have a sixth sense of what resources are available and the general stress of the organizations in which they work . . . and as resources like ventilators start to dwindle, while patients arrive in ever-increasing numbers, they will start to change what they do. As discussed at length in the next part of this book, decisions about starting life support and about withdrawal of life support are often not straightforward – particularly for the very elderly, or for patients with terminal illness. In this gray zone, the approach a physician takes can have a lot of influence. For example, a physician might say: "He's very sick and there is a chance he won't pull through, but it's not without hope – and he sounds like a fighter." Or the same physician could say: "He's very sick and chances are small. We have to think about quality of life, as well as quantity. Would he have wanted to spend the end of his life in the ICU on machines?" These differences in presentation can make big differences in the conclusions that families reach.

I suspect that in hot spots of the pandemic around the globe, in hospitals that are struggling to cope with increasing numbers of COVID-19 patients, physicians may be increasingly discouraging life support, to avoid later needing to employ explicit rationing. And I think they may actually be doing so subconsciously – because it is too painful to acknowledge directly the fact that they are, in effect, rationing. Gray areas for patients' families are also gray areas for physicians, and there are many cases in which they can convince themselves that a decision against life support is reasonable. Much like the front line in the military, the doctors on the front lines of COVID-19 in certain hot spots are suffering stress and moral injury, and are finding defense mechanisms.

Meanwhile, the lay press is making a virtue of necessity: many news articles have been published supporting the idea that ventilators are to be avoided in the setting of COVID-19 – as though they somehow cause harm, or that they signal futility. Neither is true. It's a fair question for the public to consider whether we have gone overboard in our aggressiveness in treating critical care illness in general – but COVID-19 causes illness well within the range of severity that we treat all the time, without this kind of second-guessing.

What can you do?

If you are discussing life support with your loved one's doctor during the pandemic, and you are in a hotspot where hospitals are simply overwhelmed, be aware of the existence of both explicit and "soft" rationing.

- Directly ask the doctor if she would present the decision in the same way if it were not during a pandemic, when resources are stretched. Be sympathetic, not confrontational. Your doctor may be in an untenable position.
- Ask whether the doctor would think differently about aggressiveness of care if your loved one had ARDS from a cause other than COVID-19. Remember, more and more evidence suggests that ARDS from COVID-19 behaves much like ARDS from other causes.
- Ask whether a formal organizational protocol to prioritize ventilators and ICU beds is in effect.
- Ask whether elective surgeries are still being done in the hospital (these consume anesthesia machines that could be used as ventilators).
- It is a grim reality that rationing may be necessary – but *only* in the worst crises. If you believe that decisions to withhold care are not in

your loved one's best interest – particularly if elective surgeries are still being done – request further discussion. You may even want to escalate the issue to the Chief Medical Officer (not just the COVID-19, ethics, or palliative care committees).

DEATH: COVID-19-SPECIFIC ISSUES

When patients with COVID-19 die, it may be from severe lung disease, or from complications in other organ systems – including shock from cardiac collapse and/or sepsis. As with other critical illnesses, many patients die only after the decision has been made to withdraw life support. Withdrawing life support, and what to expect, is discussed in detail in chapter 7. Remember the issue of "soft rationing" in decisions to withdraw life support, as discussed above.

Many of the issues related to dying and death are similar for all ICU patients, and are discussed in detail in chapter 7 of this book. However, there are a few issues that are specific for patients with COVID-19, and these are reviewed here.

As discussed earlier, even during and after death, visitation to your loved one with COVID-19 may not be permitted (except virtually by video conference). Outside the United States, some hospitals are beginning to permit visitors to dying COVID-19 patients, and it is my hope that restrictions will soon loosen in the United States as well. If you are permitted to visit, you should know that after death there is still the possibility that your loved one's body could transmit the infection. It is important to wear gloves and a gown when sitting with or touching your loved one after death, and to wash your hands carefully after removing gloves.

It isn't yet clear whether COVID-19 infection can be transmitted from an organ donor to someone receiving the organs. At the time of this writing, people with active COVID-19 infection cannot be organ donors. Donating the body to science (for example, for medical school anatomy courses) may still be possible for COVID-19 patients – you should check with the receiving institution, if this is something your loved one would have wanted. Autopsies can still be done (although some hospitals discourage this), and are important to our developing understanding of COVID-19.

All aspects of a normal funeral are at least in theory possible for COVID-19 patients, including embalming, open-casket viewing, cremation, and burial, as long as gloves and gown are worn when handling the body. You will want to check with individual funeral homes to understand their individual policies.

6

After the First 2 Weeks

Prolonged ICU Care and Big-Picture Decisions

Your family member has now been in the ICU for 2 weeks. What does this long stay mean for your relative's chance of recovery? You should know that long stays are common – and many patients survive to leave the hospital after *weeks or even months* in the ICU. Nonetheless, the prognosis gradually worsens a little bit with every passing day in the ICU[1] – as does the likely quality of life after discharge. Many family members of ICU patients, particularly elderly patients, begin to worry that a prolonged ICU stay would not be in accordance with their loved one's wishes. This concern tends to become an increasingly important part of the ICU experience, and of your decisions on behalf of your loved one. If you are like many people who love patients with prolonged ICU stays, you may be wondering, "When is enough enough?"

Two decisions that may need to be addressed around this time are whether your relative should have a tracheostomy and feeding tube placed (the last two procedures discussed in chapter 4 of this book). These measures are done – sometimes at the same time – with the anticipation of a long hospital course and recovery. For many family members the decision to do these procedures becomes a larger question about the patient's best interests in terms of the duration and aggressiveness of care.

This part of the book will focus on issues that have bearing on decisions about when enough is enough. *It is targeted toward those patients who remain on life support after two weeks* – seemingly in a sort of holding pattern. Life support means those treatments without which a patient would die quickly, including the mechanical ventilator, and medications or devices needed to maintain an adequate blood pressure (usually those who need the latter also need a mechanical ventilator). If your loved one is not currently on life support, then he is likely moving toward discharge from the ICU, and making decisions about when enough is enough are not as acutely relevant. You may prefer to skip to another part of the book. Similarly, if you feel these questions are not relevant for your loved one despite being on prolonged life support, feel free to skip ahead.

"HOW COULD I EVEN THINK ABOUT GIVING UP?"

This question was asked of me once by a patient's daughter, with tears in her eyes. Her elderly mother had been in the ICU on life support for more than two weeks, and I had proposed a tracheostomy and feeding tube in anticipation of a very long course of care. The daughter was beginning to wonder whether all this was what her mother would have wanted, or even in her best interest. As her mother's decision-maker, she was considering withdrawing life support – but she felt guilty for even considering giving up the fight. After all, wasn't her mother engaged in the fight of her life? Didn't she need her daughter to fight with her? This young woman was unusually courageous in asking the question aloud, but I think many people with loved ones on prolonged life support have just the same question very much in mind.

It is important to know that decisions about withdrawing life support are not monstrous – to the contrary, they are a common and necessary result of just how terribly good the ICU has become at keeping people alive. With machines to take over the work of the lungs, heart, and kidneys, and with medications to control blood pressure and fluid and electrolyte balance, we can now keep almost *anyone* technically "alive" – way past the point that it makes sense, in that they could return to reasonable quality of life. No one wants that for their loved one. When people die in the ICU, it is usually *not* because they die despite the machines and medications. Sixty-five percent of the deaths that occur in the ICU occur after a decision to withdraw care.[2] We must recognize that family members are frequently obliged to help make decisions about when "enough is enough."

We all die eventually. At some point, the most important question becomes not *whether* we will die, but how. When the time is right, shifting to the latter question is the most courageous and loving thing you can do for the patient. You should know that your loved one (or his proxy, if your relative is not able to make decisions) *always* has the right to refuse care or request that care be withdrawn – including life support such as a mechanical ventilator, blood pressure medications, and tube feeds. You should also know that if that decision is made, your relative can be kept completely comfortable – without pain or shortness of breath – while his life ends. This is discussed in more detail in the section "A comfortable death," in chapter 7.

If you are the medical decision-maker, it can feel like a terrible responsibility to decide to withdraw life support. But you should remember that it is not actually your job to make your own independent decision. Your job is to represent *what you think your family member would want*, as best as you can. In fact, this might be quite different from what you yourself think is best. Making end-of-life decisions for loved ones sometimes requires great selflessness.

You should also realize that while your judgment is important, the physician also carries responsibility. How that responsibility is shouldered differs a lot by individual, country, and generation. Older generations of doctors trained in a paternalistic era in which physicians were strongly directive in end-of-life decision-making. Some countries have cultures that still promote a more paternalistic approach (for example, France). Younger physicians in the United States trained when patient autonomy was emphasized, and are more welcoming to family participation in decision-making. In fact, I believe younger doctors will sometimes use respect for patient autonomy as an excuse to abdicate responsibility for difficult decisions altogether. Some international researchers feel that the United States produces a great deal of post-traumatic stress disorder by asking family members to make painful decisions about withdrawing life support.[3] But despite the traumatic nature of such decisions, a survey of U.S. family members found that 86 percent say that they *want* to take on that responsibility.[4]

Problems arise when family members and doctors have discordant views of their roles – for example, when the family wants to help make the decision, but doctors aren't receptive to that; or when the family wants to leave the decision-making primarily to the doctor, but the doctor refuses to take that role.[4] It may be helpful to explain to your physician explicitly what you want your role to be. If you feel she isn't taking enough responsibility for the decision, consider saying something like, "This really feels like an impossible decision for us to make, doctor. Now that you have listened to what we've told you, we'd be grateful if you told us what you think the right decision would be, if this were your family member." If your loved one's doctor *isn't* allowing the proxy to be part of decision-making, that's even more difficult to deal with. You could say something to the effect of, "It's helpful to know your view. But my understanding is that ultimately I need to make the decision as the legal representative – isn't that correct?" If you feel she is still not adequately receptive to input from family, ask to speak with a patient advocate or the hospital ethics committee.

AVERAGE PROGNOSIS FOR PATIENTS
ON PROLONGED LIFE SUPPORT

The first thing you will want to know when you consider when enough is enough is the likely outcome of the ICU admission. What are the chances that – if you keep up this long, hard struggle – your relative will survive, and survive with an acceptable quality of life? The starting place is to consider what happens to the "average" patient on prolonged life support – recognizing, of course, that no one patient is truly average.

In terms of surviving long enough to eventually be discharged from the hospital, even after two weeks of mechanical ventilation, the odds are in your family member's favor: about two-thirds of patients requiring prolonged life support survive. But what about quality of life? If your relative gets out of the hospital, chances are he will be in for a heck of a year, as I will discuss in detail below. I don't want to be too discouraging – as you will read, if your loved one survives and makes it through the long difficult recovery, there is a decent chance of recovering a good life. But anyone making decisions for someone on prolonged life support should understand that the ICU is only the first part of what is likely a very long haul. In my opinion, this is at least as important to consider as survival, when making decisions about when enough is enough.

What do I mean by a "heck of a year"? First of all, fewer than 1 in 6 patients who have prolonged mechanical ventilation in the ICU are discharged from the hospital to their home – the rest are initially discharged to some kind of skilled nursing, rehabilitation, or long-term care facility. Increasingly, patients are discharged from ICUs while they are still on a mechanical ventilator, to specialized ventilator weaning facilities. Moreover, over the course of the year, they will be moved between various care locations an average of about four times – and most will require at least one readmission to the hospital. These patients will spend most of the year either in a health care facility, or receiving paid care at home.[5]

All of this assumes they survive the year. *Only about two-thirds of patients who leave the ICU after prolonged ventilation do survive this first difficult year.* Those who survive often experience persistent physical disabilities, and dependency on caregivers. At one year after the ICU stay, 2 in 5 surviving patients have difficulty with bladder and bowel control *and* are dependent on others for help with all of the following activities of daily living: bathing, dressing, feeding, toileting, and moving from bed to chair. Fewer than 1 in 5 are completely independent.[4] Many have persistent problems with their thinking or memory, and/or psychological problems like depression and post-traumatic stress disorder (PTSD).[6] Those who were in the ICU with severe lung disease, such as ARDS, may have some degree of shortness of breath for as long as 5 years,[7] although eventually this typically resolves completely.

The pie chart (figure 6.1) shows the outcomes for patients discharged from the hospital after prolonged mechanical ventilation, one year after their discharge.

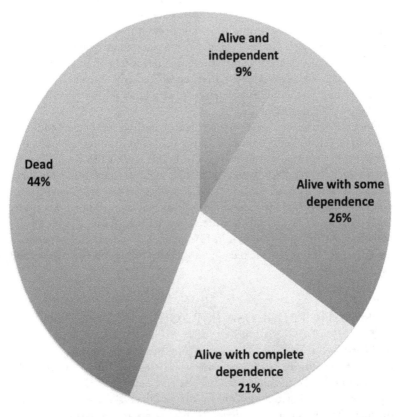

Figure 6.1. How do people do after prolonged mechanical ventilation? Outcomes one year after leaving the ICU. *Source*: Adapted from data from Unroe et al., "One-year trajectories of care and resource utilization for recipients of prolonged mechanical ventilation: A cohort study," *Annals of Internal Medicine* 153, no. 3 (2010): 167–175.

Notes: Complete dependence means needing help with all of the following activities: bathing, dressing, feeding, transferring from bed to chair, bladder and bowel control, and use of toilet. Some dependence means needing help with 1–5 of these activities.

The good news is that in subsequent years, things start to look up. The two-thirds of ICU survivors who are strong enough to make it past this one-year hurdle tend to do pretty well in terms of getting back quality of life and independence – almost all 3-year survivors, for example, are independent and living at home.[8] But it is important that you understand that your loved one isn't out of the woods by any means after leaving the ICU, and even if he survives, there is likely a long road ahead. Often, this isn't explained well to patients' families, and they have no idea just how fraught and difficult the coming year is likely to be. For example, when asked about their predictions for ICU patients one year after discharge, family members are more than twice as likely as their ICU doctors to expect that their loved one will be alive, more than 10 times as likely to expect that their loved one will be without major deficiencies in functioning, and more than 20 times as likely to think that their loved one will have a good quality of life.[9]

On an uplifting note, even those patients who have the longest and most grueling experiences after admission to the ICU tend to say in retrospect that they are glad they were put on life support. In one study, patients who were on prolonged mechanical ventilation (in the ICU and subsequently in a ventilator weaning facility) were asked six months later whether they would have chosen again to go through the process of mechanical ventilation. The large majority (85%) said yes.[10] To me, this is a touching tribute to people's extraordinary resilience and inherent good nature. However, I can't help but suspect that it's also partly because of the memory loss associated with both sedatives and psychological trauma.

SPECIFIC PROGNOSIS FOR YOUR FAMILY MEMBER

It's all very well to talk about the average experience for patients requiring prolonged life support. But individual patients vary widely. What about *your* relative, specifically? For example, will *your* relative be among the few who survive and go home quickly to a good quality of life? Or, possibly, will he be among the few who have devastating disability many years after discharge? After all, these are the kind of questions that are most relevant to your decision about when enough is enough. Surely, with all that is known about your relative medically at this point, it ought to be possible to give a confident prognosis.

But unfortunately, this may not be the case. For patients at the extreme ends of the spectrum – those who are exceedingly sick, and those who are really quite well – ICU doctors have a pretty good idea of what will happen. But for the majority of patients who fall in the gray zone between the extremes, the fact is that we are just not very good at predicting outcomes.

Of course, we have a general idea about what characteristics make it more likely a patient will have worse outcomes – for example: old age; a medical reason for being in the ICU (rather than a surgical reason such as trauma); and the diagnoses of metastatic cancer, ARDS, septic shock, or ICU delirium. We also have an array of predictive scores at our disposal, which are calculated based on data like vital signs and lab results, as well as the presence of chronic illnesses. Examples of these measures are the acute physiology and chronic health evaluation (APACHE), mortality probability model (MPM), and sequential organ failure assessment (SOFA) scores. These scores are generally calculated at the time of admission or over the first couple of days, and generate an estimate of the probability of death. For example, a patient admitted with gastrointestinal bleeding and a rapid heart rate, low blood pressure, acute kidney problems, and respiratory failure has a predicted mortality of 47.7 percent, according to the Mortality Probability Model (MPM). However, despite the precision implied by the decimal point, such scores are notoriously unreliable, and will not be very helpful to you. While they are useful for research and measuring the severity of critical illness in populations, they are too uncertain for predicting outcomes in individual patients. Because for many ICU patients it is so difficult to predict outcomes, you may well get different answers from different caretakers[11] – which can be frustrating and upsetting.

I can speak to this prognostic uncertainty on a personal level. As a very young ICU physician, I felt fairly confident – too confident – of my predictive abilities. But it only took a few years of practice to rack up a number of cases with outcomes that surprised me. I will never forget one elderly patient who had been in the ICU on mechanical ventilation for almost two months after requiring emergency surgery on his aorta (the giant artery sending blood from the heart). The surgery had been complicated by an infection, sepsis, and multi-organ failure, and he had had a long and difficult ICU course. He had just acquired the most recent of many complications during his ICU stay: an infection of his central line, with recurrent sepsis, shock, and kidney failure. I scheduled a late afternoon meeting with the family, at which time I planned to tell them I thought there was almost no chance of survival, and that I recommended considering withdrawing life support. This family trusted me, and they were at the end of their rope – I have no doubt they would have followed my advice. But at the last minute, a colleague pointed out to me that I was very tired (I had gotten almost no sleep the previous night, and had had a frantically busy day). He reminded me that this was not the kind of decision to make, or conversation to have, while exhausted. I postponed the meeting.

The next morning, some of my patient's lab results and vital signs were just a *smidge* better. I still didn't think there was a chance he would survive, but I decided to put off the meeting another day. And then another.

Five months later, this same gentleman was sending me a postcard from a resort where he was playing golf, to say hello and to thank me again for his care. I've had similar experiences where patients came back seemingly from the brink of certain death, and others where patients I thought would do well did not. It doesn't take many experiences like this to make you very humble, and cautious in your predictions. If your doctor tells you she isn't sure what will happen to your loved one, she isn't necessarily being evasive. She may just be unusually honest.

THE TYRANNY OF HOPE

So if it is so difficult to predict survival and other outcomes for many ICU patients – how on earth are families and doctors to make good decisions for patients? It is hard enough to make the agonizing decisions about when enough is enough, without this uncertainty.

Once, when I was training to be an ICU doctor, I expressed frustration to a very smart member of my faculty about our profession's inability to accurately assess patients' prognoses (likely outcomes). He thought for a while and said, "I'm not sure it matters."

"Why on earth wouldn't that matter?" I asked, a little exasperated.

"Say you could accurately predict a bad outcome. Say you could confidently say to a patient's family, 'I am sure that this patient has a 97 percent chance of dying, despite all our heroics and weeks on life support.'"

"OK, wouldn't that be important to that family, in terms of making decisions about withdrawing care?"

He scratched his head. "Maybe for a few families. But nine times out of ten, families are going to say, 'OK, let's take that chance. Let's go for the 3 percent odds. It's worth it if we can save him.' So maybe it doesn't matter so much for us to be able to say accurately, it's a 75 percent chance of death versus a 97 percent chance of death."

Dr. Rubenfeld was referring to what I later came to think of as the *tyranny of hope*. For the sake of very small chances for a good outcome, many family members are willing to go through hell and back. The inevitable consequence of this "long odds" strategy is that many patients end up on the losing end, receiving weeks of aggressive care that didn't benefit them and caused unnecessary suffering. It is similar to a casino. A few players may win big, but on the whole the odds favor the casino owners.

As Dr. Atul Gawande, physician and author, says about end-of-life decisions: "Hope is not a plan."[12]

TWO APPROACHES TO MAKING END-OF-LIFE DECISIONS

I've come to realize that there are two broad, very different approaches to making decisions for loved ones about when enough is enough. If you are the proxy, which approach you should take depends on the medical and life circumstances of your relative, as well as on his personality.

The first is the *"long odds" approach* described above, in which small hopes for survival become the most important factor. There is no doubt that this will be the most appropriate strategy in some cases – where hope is, in fact, the best plan. For example, imagine a young woman, previously in good health, who is on prolonged life support after a devastating car accident. She has three school-age children at home, including one with a learning disability. She might well want to keep fighting no matter what she has to go through, and no matter how vanishingly small the chances. Or imagine a middle-aged man who has gone through a bone marrow transplant for leukemia and now has an infection. He has shown himself over the years to be a tireless fighter, remaining hungry for every moment life can give him.

For some patients, it may be better to use a very different strategy. This second strategy – which I will call the *"most likely scenario" approach* – ignores the temptation of small hopes and focuses on the scenario that is most probable for the patient. For example, consider a very elderly gentleman who has had a rich and accomplished life. He has remarked to his wife on many occasions that although he loves his life, he feels he has lived it fully, and is at peace with the idea of death. Imagine that his doctors estimate he has a 20 percent chance of survival with meaningful quality of life. The young woman with three children might well want to take those odds, but for this gentleman it might be more important to consider the most likely scenario: what is *probable* (at an 80 percent likelihood) is that he goes through a long, difficult hospital course only to die, or to survive with a miserable quality of life. A family member, knowing the patient's values, might take the "most likely scenario" approach and decide that continued aggressive care was not appropriate for this man.

What about your relative? Based on what you know about him, which approach is most appropriate? Do you think your loved one would want you to set your sights on small chances, or do you feel you can best answer your responsibility to your loved one by planning based on what is *most likely?* Explicitly choosing between these two very different strategies – "long odds" or "most likely scenario"—may help to provide some clarity as you make your decisions.

PERSONALITY CHARACTERISTICS

Usually, when given the same information, most people would agree about what was best. For example, in my experience, most elderly people with end-stage cancer and poor functional status even before ICU admission would not want prolonged life support in the ICU. Most young, previously healthy people in the ICU because of a car accident (without significant brain injury) *would* want prolonged life support. However, there are important exceptions where particular personality characteristics become very important, and might lead a person to make an unusual decision. In some cases, reasonable people might disagree.

I remember one such case. Mr. Pagano was a 71-year-old man with underlying lung disease from many years of smoking, who had been admitted with pneumonia and sepsis. He had recovered from his infection, but because of his lung disease we had not been able to get him off his mechanical ventilator, after weeks of trying. He had just developed a catheter-associated urinary tract infection with a relatively drug-resistant bacteria, recurrent sepsis, and delirium. I thought we could probably treat the infection with broad-spectrum antibiotics, but at best it would set him back at least another week. His most likely course, if he recovered from the urinary tract infection, was to be discharged to a ventilator weaning facility for several weeks. If he was successfully weaned of the ventilator and did not develop further complications, he could anticipate a long stay in a rehabilitation unit. It was quite possible he would require care in a facility or paid home care for months or even years, and that he might not ever be fully independent again. In fact, there was a chance he might never be free of the ventilator.

During his long admission, I had come to know Mr. Pagano a little indirectly, through interaction with his family. I knew he was a first-generation Italian immigrant who had worked hard to build a new life for himself and his family in the United States, and my impression was that he was a man of strength and perseverance. I decided to have a meeting with the family to discuss his options (at the time he was not competent to make his own decisions). In the course of the discussion, what also emerged was that Mr. Pagano prized his independence above almost anything else. His daughter said that although Mr. Pagano had extremely poor eyesight, throughout his life he had refused to wear glasses because he saw it as an unacceptable sign of weakness. In that moment, I was pretty sure I knew what Mr. Pagano would want. How would a man who couldn't accept the help of glasses tolerate being bedridden for months, years, or possibly forever – fully dependent on those around him for even the simplest needs and personal care?

After a long discussion about Mr. Pagano, his medical situation, and the likely outcomes, the family decided to wait and see if his delirium would subside enough in the next few days that they could discuss the options with him. However, he remained unable to discuss his options the next week, and at that point the family made the loving decision to withdraw life support.

Fierce independence is one important personality characteristic that, in my experience, frequently affects patients' and families' decisions about when enough is enough. Another personality characteristic is the need to be physically fit and active. For some people, the idea of being bed-bound is intolerable (while for others, it is a chance to read a good book).

Another is being deeply religious. Often, devout families are concerned about withdrawing life support because they believe it is against God's will. However, it could equally well be argued that keeping someone alive through artificial means and machines is working against God's plan. As I once heard a Mormon physician telling his Mormon patient's wife, "When God is pulling him by the hands, who are we to hang on to his heels?"

THE TENDENCY TOWARD OPTIMISM

The tendency toward optimism is found in doctors and families alike, and mutually reinforced. One study showed that almost two-thirds of doctors overestimated the duration of their terminally ill patients' survival – on average by a factor of five.[13]

But family members are even more prone to be optimistic. I have already told you about the research that shows that family members are much more likely than ICU doctors to believe patients will survive, be independent, and have a good quality of life after they leave the ICU. Almost certainly, part of this is a failure of ICU staff to communicate realistic expectations[14] (perhaps because they are trying to be kind, and to not crush hope).

However, it's also been shown that *even when given the information*, family members tend to see it with rose-colored glasses – particularly when it's bad news. For example, in one study, when family members were explicitly told the patient had a 5 percent chance of survival, they came away from the conversation believing that the chance of survival was three times higher.[15] Often, such family members believe that patient attributes unknown to the physician will lead to better-than-predicted outcomes – for example, that the patient has always been "a fighter" with a strong will to live. They may also have the superstitious (and sometimes subconscious) belief that their own outlook and capacity for hope will in some way influence the outcome.

You should be on the lookout for this tendency toward optimism in yourself and other family members. There is nothing wrong with hoping for the best, but you can't let it cloud your judgment when your relative is relying on your decisions.

A BEAUTIFUL END

"So we beat on, boats against the current, borne back ceaselessly into the past."

—F. Scott Fitzgerald

Because of our ability to keep people alive long after it makes sense, decisions about withdrawing life support are necessary and common. But they are not algorithmic: they are more art than science, and intensely personal. Everyone wrestles with how best to approach them – including your doctors. Certainly, including me. In this section, I'll share my own thoughts on the matter as they have developed over time.

By way of background, a patient's son and I were once discussing whether to take the "long-odds approach" and continue aggressive care for his father – who had a *very* small chance of surviving. His son asked me whether his father was comfortable. I told him that I thought he was (he was deeply sedated). The son asked me earnestly, "Then why *not* push forward as hard and long as possible? If he isn't feeling or aware of any of this, what's the downside?"

I thought long and hard about this question, many years after it was asked of me. First of all, although most very sick ICU patients are kept largely free of pain and are often asleep, it is almost impossible to fully avoid moments of shortness of breath, panic, confusion, nightmares, and discomfort – and most ICU patients will later remember some of these.[16] But what also seems important to me are the indignities and the sadness of the patients' situations – regardless of whether they are conscious of them.

What do I mean by indignities and sadness? ICU patients have no control and are wholly dependent on others for care and decisions. They usually can't communicate meaningfully with the people who are close to them. They are removed from the context and surroundings that give them their identity, unknown among caretakers who are essentially strangers. Their bodies are often exposed, with no ability to protect modesty. They are surrounded 24 hours a day by plastic and machinery, bright lights, and noise.

But the worst insult to these patients may be the effect on their own loved ones. I've watched many families who spend weeks or months in the ICU. In the early days, the room is full and alive with questions, talk, tears, reassurances, and people coming and going. But over time, the atmosphere becomes more solemn and quiet. Toward the end, fewer family members come. Those closest to the patient sit propped pale and motionless against the wall, exhausted and numb – beaten down by their experience and their grief. Eventually, family members may reach the point where they decide to withdraw life support. But the decision sometimes carries the feeling of an abject surrender. My heart aches for these families, and also for the patients – who would not have wanted their families to go through this ordeal on their account.

These were the images that flooded my head when my patient's son asked, "Why *not* push forward as hard and long as possible?" What I didn't say was that, *for your father's sake, I don't want to see you beaten down in this way.*

In college I majored in English and American literature. When I decided, late, to go to medical school, my area of study sure seemed like it had been a wrong turn – but ironically, I now call on it to understand my feelings about end-of-life decisions as an ICU doctor. As any English major knows, the most important part of any book or poem is the ending – the last line or paragraph. F. Scott Fitzgerald's *The Great Gatsby*; Annie Proulx's *The Shipping News*; Gerard Manley Hopkins' *Spring and Fall*; Yann Martel's *Life of Pi*; Zora Neale Hurston's *Their Eyes Were Watching God*; William Butler Yeats' *Sailing to Byzantium* . . . how much less would any of these works have been without the impact of their ending?

I realize that I have come to believe that a life should be like any other great work: it should have a beautiful ending. Everyone deserves that chance at a strong and graceful closure. What is a beautiful ending, for a human? That will differ depending on who you ask. But one thing I think we would all agree on: it is not the situation of indignities and sadness that I described earlier.

I believe I have seen beautiful endings happen many times, even in the ICU. To me, such a death includes:

1. Dignity and control: The patient (or patient's proxy) accepts death and makes intentional decisions about how and when it happens.

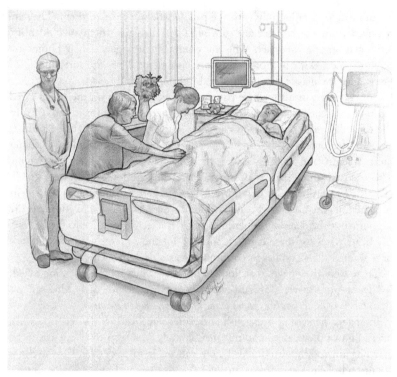

Figure 6.2.   A beautiful end © 2021 Laurie O'Keefe

2. Family closeness: The patient's family is harmonious and brought closer by the situation. Family members take time at the bedside to say good-byes and express love and appreciation.

3. Family well-being: The family has not been beaten down into a state of submission and exhaustion by the ICU ordeal.

4. Grief: Grief is a good thing: it is on the other side of the coin from love. The saddest deaths are those where there is no one grieving – either because the patient has no one close to him, or because the family is too numb and exhausted.

5. Compassion: The patient is kept completely comfortable, even if the necessary sedatives hasten death.

6. Respectful atmosphere: Tubes and wires are removed wherever possible, the patient is covered to protect modesty, the room is arranged for family comfort, alarms are turned off, and staff interruptions are minimized.

Not everyone thinks as I do about the value of a beautiful end. I remember one daughter (a well-educated and very smart lawyer) who was angry with me when I told her my view. This isn't about aesthetics, she told me. This is about whether my father lives or dies.

I couldn't argue. But for me it is about both.

What can you do?

1. If you are the medical decision-maker, understand that your job is not to decide what *you* want for the patient, but to represent what you think the *patient* would want – based on all you know of him, and conversations you may have had.

2. Recognize that it is often necessary to make decisions about when "enough is enough," and that these decisions are courageous and loving. At some point the important question becomes *how* a person dies, rather than *whether* a person dies.

3. Try to understand your relative's likely prognosis, as best you can. Ask your doctor if there is "almost no hope" of survival – or, at the other extreme, if she's fairly certain that your family member will recover. Understand that between these extremes, it is very difficult for your doctor to predict the future.

4. Quality of life is as important as survival. Ask your doctor about how she envisions your loved one six months or a year from now. Is your loved one likely to be home? Likely to be dependent on others for daily activities?

5. Decide which approach to decision-making makes most sense for your loved one, given the particular circumstances. Should you take the "long-odds" approach? Or is it instead your responsibility to plan based on what is "most likely"?

6. Next, consider your loved one's personality and how it might affect his wishes. For example, consider how easily your loved one could accept being dependent on others or physically inactive.

7. End-of-life decisions are best made through a partnership between families and doctors. Your doctor needs to hear from you what circumstances and personal characteristics are important, and what you think the patient would want. You need to hear from your doctor about the medical situation and prognosis. You might want to ask your doctor, "What would you do if this were your family member?"

7

Dying in the ICU

This chapter of the book is for you in the unfortunate event that your family member is in the 10–20 percent of patients who do not survive to leave the ICU. *If your family member is not in the dying process or about to have life support discontinued, you will probably want to skip this chapter.*

No one hopes to die in the ICU. Most people in the United States say they would like to die at home. However, only about a third of people actually do die at home, and about the same number die in a hospital[1] – often after an ICU stay. When people say they hope to die at home, they also presumably hope to die quickly and peacefully, without discomfort, and without causing undue distress or burden for family members. But this isn't always the way it happens. In the ICU, at least, it is possible to make sure that death is comfortable, and to take some of the burden from family members so that they are able to focus on saying goodbye to their loved one. If your loved one must die in the ICU, the goal is to bring as many advantages of a home death as possible to his bedside.

In this chapter of the book, I'll discuss what death means physically. I'll talk about what you should do to prepare if you know death is coming, including considering organ donation. I'll then discuss what exactly you can expect during the dying process, and how your ICU caregivers will ensure a comfortable death. Finally, I'll describe some of the logistical matters and decisions that arise after death.

HOW DO PEOPLE DIE IN THE ICU,
AND WHAT IS DEATH?

Most people in the ICU die after the withdrawal of life support – for example, the mechanical ventilator, or medications and devices necessary to maintain adequate blood pressure. Some people die despite continuation of life support and aggressive measures. These patients generally have catastrophic failure of their lungs, heart, and circulatory system, requiring unsuccessful rounds of cardiopulmonary resuscitation. The irreversible failure of the heart and lungs to sustain the critical functions of the body is called circulatory death. After a few minutes, circulatory death inevitably causes brain death, because the brain is not getting adequate blood flow and oxygen.

Sometimes, brain death occurs without circulatory death, after a severe neurologic injury (from trauma, asphyxiation, or brief cardiac arrest, for example). It is important to recognize that brain death is different from coma. Coma is a state of profoundly impaired consciousness, and is sometimes reversible. However, brain death is the *permanent* loss of all functions of the brain. In the case of suspected brain death, the doctor will often do a special neurologic exam, including a test of whether the patient makes any respiratory effort. (Out of an abundance of caution, some doctors will repeat this exam after an interval ranging from a few hours to a couple of days.) A patient who is brain dead is legally considered dead. This can be counterintuitive, because breathing can be artificially continued with the ventilator, and the heart may continue to beat. But the patient is indeed irreversibly dead, and life support must be withdrawn.

WHEN YOU KNOW DEATH IS COMING

In some cases, you will have advance warning that death is imminent. This is particularly true if the decision has been made to withdraw life support. In this case, there are a few things you may want to do in preparation. If possible, delegate these tasks to other family members or friends. They are looking for ways to help.

What can you do if death is imminent?

- Look through your loved one's papers for a "letter of instruction" about wishes for after-death arrangements; prearrangements for funeral services; documentation of wishes about organ donation (for example, on a driver's license); or contracts with medical institutions for donation of the body to science.

- Inform the people closest to you and to your loved one (but clearly specify whether they should or should not come to the hospital).
- There are many arrangements to be made after death. If you feel that you will not be in a state of mind to handle these, ask one of the people close to you if they will be the point person to help you.
- Bring in any photos, music, or personal items you would like to have in the room during your loved one's death.
- Consider organ donation (discussed below).

PLANNING AHEAD: ORGAN DONATION

The decision to donate organs is a complicated one. Those who have made this decision have done an incredibly generous and important thing. The science of transplanting organs has advanced tremendously, and we can now offer years of high-quality life to people who otherwise would have died. A single donor can save up to eight lives and improve many more, through donations of the heart, lungs, liver, kidneys, pancreas, intestines, bone, corneas, and skin. More than 100,000 patients – including young people and children – are desperately awaiting donor organs, and almost 20 of them die daily because no organs are available.[2]

The decision to donate organs should ideally be made before a patient's heart and breathing stop, although some organs may still be donated if the decision is made quickly after death. If the decision is delayed too long, the organs will no longer be viable. Often, the decision to donate is made when the patient is still on life support, but has been diagnosed with brain death (for example, after a severe head injury), or the decision has been made to withdraw life support for another reason.

Your loved one may have already made the decision to be an organ donor, before being admitted to the ICU. His driver's license may indicate this, or he may be listed in your state registry. Hospital staff can contact an organ donor coordinator who will be able to confirm this for you. If your loved one has previously recorded a decision about organ donation, this is legally binding and can't be overturned by the proxy or family members, unless the patient is a minor (under 18 years old). If your loved one has not previously recorded a decision about organ donation, the proxy may do so. If you are the proxy, remember that the question is *not* how you feel about your loved one giving organs – but what you think he would have wanted. For many patients and families, donating organs is a way to make something positive come out of a deeply sad event.

Old age, infection (including sepsis and hepatitis), and cancer do not necessarily preclude donation. Even if some organs are not usable, others may be. Don't assume that your loved one cannot be an organ donor without first speaking with an organ donation coordinator.

Federal regulations require that hospitals notify the local organ procurement organization (OPO) about all imminent deaths. An OPO coordinator will then do an initial screen to see if the patient is registered as an organ donor, and if he meets initial criteria for eligibility. If so, the coordinator will meet with the family to discuss organ donation, and to obtain authorization from the proxy (if the patient has not previously given authorization). Care is taken to separate the responsibilities of the clinical staff from the OPO, to minimize even the appearance of a conflict of interest (in which, for example, the doctors encourage withdrawing life support in order to "get" the organs). The clinical staff's responsibility is always to think about the best interests and medical care of the patient. Your doctors and nurses are expected to leave detailed conversations about organ donation to the OPO coordinator, and in many cases, the OPO coordinator may be the first person to raise the topic with the family.

If your loved one or the proxy does authorize organ donation, the OPO will then direct an in-depth evaluation of whether the patient is a suitable donor, and if so, for what organs. Certain procedures may be necessary to evaluate the health and suitability of the organs – for example, blood tests, bronchoscopy to inspect the lungs and exclude pneumonia, and biopsy of the liver.

After death, organs are procured in the operating room. The patient's surgical incisions are closed, just as after any surgery. Organ donation does not interfere with an open-casket funeral.

It is so very hard even to think beyond your loved one's death, let alone think about something as invasive to his person as organ donation. But doing so is quite literally life-saving. I can't think of a more generous act or powerful legacy for you and your loved one to leave.

What can you do?

- Check your loved one's driver's license and the state registry to see if he is an organ donor. Hospital staff can help you with this.

- If you are the proxy, remember that your responsibility is to decide whether your loved one would have wanted to donate organs – putting your own feelings and beliefs aside.
- If you think your loved one would want to be an organ donor and it seems likely that his death is imminent over the next day or two, confirm with your doctor that the local Organ Procurement Organization (OPO) has been contacted, and ask to speak with an organ donation coordinator.
- Your physician and other ICU team members are expected to focus on the best medical care of your loved one, independent of decisions about organ donation. In many cases, they are not expert in questions such as suitability for organ donation. The OPO coordinator is your best and most appropriate source of information about donation.

WITHDRAWING LIFE SUPPORT: WHAT TO EXPECT

Most people who die in the ICU do so after a decision to withdraw life support. Should you stay with your loved one during this process? This is another difficult decision. In most cases, at least one or two family members stay. For some family members it may be just too hard. But I think that if you are an adult and can find the strength to be there, you will be glad. For your loved one, you may be able to provide comfort and company. For yourself, you may take comfort in having been close and present until the very end.

If you are the proxy, you may want to restrict the people in the room to just those closest to your loved one, or even just to yourself. Like childbirth, this is an intimate moment, possibly meant only for the inner circle. If you or your loved one is religious, you may want to ask for a chaplain, rabbi, or other clergy to visit (many hospitals have clergy on site).

It is my belief that it helps a great deal if you know exactly what to expect when life support is discontinued. The following paragraphs explain exactly what will happen, including how your loved one may look and act. Some of these changes are distressing (especially if unexpected), but you should know that they are part of the dying process and don't necessarily indicate pain or discomfort. *If you have decided not to be in the room or just don't want to learn about these things right now, you should skip ahead to the next section.*

First, the nurse will discontinue medications (except for sedatives and pain medications), tube feedings, and intravenous fluids. If your relative has required large amounts of fluids or blood pressure medications, you may see the blood pressure reading on the monitor quickly fall to lower levels. Now it is time to remove ventilator support. Your nurse may give your relative a large amount of a sedative first, to prevent shortness of breath. The ventilator may be simply turned off, or sometimes the amount of work it does is rapidly reduced over the course of about 30–60 minutes, until it is no longer providing any support. During that time, sedatives will be given as needed to treat shortness of breath. Finally, the endotracheal tube will be removed.

Tubes, lines, and gear will be removed, whenever possible. Alarms on the IV pumps and monitors in the room will ideally be silenced.

How long will it take for your loved one to die? This is another area in which doctors are terrible at making predictions. It is so distressing to patients' families when their expectations are wrong that I hesitate to give a specific prediction for most patients. However, it is important to understand the possible range.[3] If the patient is in catastrophic circulatory collapse, it may take only minutes. In most cases, it takes about an hour. However, in about a quarter of cases it takes more than several hours – and very rarely, it can take days. If the dying process is continuing more than a few hours and the ICU bed is needed by an incoming patient, your relative might be transferred to a non-ICU room in the hospital. The idea of such transfers is understandably distressing to families – but there is a silver lining: it usually means a quieter, nicer room.

What can you expect during this time? Your relative may breathe shallowly and slowly, and it may be noisy. In a state of deep unconsciousness, the neck muscles around the airway relax, and saliva and sputum accumulate, creating turbulent air flow and sounds. As the dying process continues, there may be a breathing pattern that looks like intermittent breathing (with groups of fast breaths alternating with groups of slow breaths), and ultimately, infrequent breaths or gasping. Remember that slow gasping in this setting does not in itself signal discomfort. Sometimes, breathing may appear to stop completely, even for a minute or two, and family at the bedside may believe the patient has died – but then there is one last gasp. This can be disconcerting, particularly if you aren't prepared for it.

There are other physical changes to expect. Your relative's skin may become cool, dusky purple, or mottled, because of changes in blood flow and oxygen levels. In the final moments, your loved one may have jerking movements of the head, arms, legs, or abdomen. These are spinal reflexes that can occur even after brain death. One such reflex involves pulling the arms up across the chest. Like the last breath, such movements can be startling. Remember that they are part of the dying process, and don't mean that your loved one is uncomfortable.

How should you be during this process? Surely this is your ultimate test. Try to put the physical changes out of your mind. Try not to focus obsessively on the heartbeat on the monitor (you can ask your nurse to turn off the monitor display, if you prefer). This is not a time to be distracted by details, but to focus on honoring and being present with your loved one. Reflect on who he is, and his life. Hold his hand and talk to him. Tell him whatever is important or as yet unsaid. We do not know how much someone can hear or process during final moments, but my guess is that your relative might find comfort in your company and the sound of your voice.

You may not be sure what to say. There may be so much to say that it feels overwhelming to start. My advice is just to start, even if the words don't feel adequate at first. I have observed that once family members begin to talk to a dying loved one, the floodgates open and it is suddenly clear what needs to be said.

A COMFORTABLE DEATH

Your family member can and should be kept completely comfortable during the dying process. We have powerful medications that can eradicate pain and shortness of breath. (Just to illustrate the point, we regularly use such medications to put people to sleep before major surgery, quite successfully.) There is absolutely no reason and no justification for providing inadequate sedation and pain control.

These medications will drop blood pressure and slow breathing – so they will hasten death. But remember that the question has shifted from whether and when the person dies, to *how* he dies – and the single most important factor is that death be painless and peaceful. You should have complete clarity about this.

I am sorry to say that not all medical personnel have complete clarity. A few may feel uneasy about delivering large amounts of medications that will hasten death. To alleviate this unease, many doctors and nurses adhere to an old theological doctrine called the "principle of double effect." In the context of health care, it holds sedatives are justifiable, even if they hasten death, if the *primary intent* is to alleviate discomfort. Thus, hastening death is an unintended secondary consequence. In my experience, one of the practical problems with the principle of double effect is that it requires the patient to demonstrate discomfort before caretakers increase sedation. Since sedation takes a minute or two to take effect, you can get unacceptably behind while chasing symptoms. There are certain situations when discomfort can be anticipated (for example, shortness of breath after discontinuing the mechanical ventilator in some patients). In these situations, sedatives are needed even before there is a pressing need, to *prevent* discomfort. In addition, many physicians and nurses feel that concerns about hastening death become specious and counterproductive past a certain point in the dying process.

You can play an important role in ensuring your relative's comfort by demonstrating your own clarity about the priority of ensuring comfort. Let your nurses and doctors know that this is your primary concern. Several minutes before the ventilator is withdrawn, ask the nurse if she will give a dose of morphine or another sedative, to prevent any shortness of breath. Give the nurse constant feedback about how you think your relative is doing. Moaning, restlessness, or rapid breathing may be signs of discomfort. (As described above, noisy and irregular breathing is to be expected – but if the patient is comfortable, the respiratory rate is usually normal or slow.) When in doubt about whether the patient is uncomfortable, err on the side of "yes." Use the code phrase "I think he looks uncomfortable"; this gives the nurse permission and justification to increase sedatives, if she is operating under the principle of double effect. After all, you will be far more attuned and sensitive to your loved one's experience than his caretakers.

What can you do?

- Decide who will be in the room during the death (for example, adults who are in the closest inner circle). If you can't bear to be there, that is okay. But if you find the strength to be there through the end, I think you will be glad.
- Know what to expect. Review with the doctor and nurse exactly what steps will be taken in what order, and how they expect it to go.
- Tell your caregivers clearly that your number one priority is that your family member stays comfortable, even if that hastens death. Tell your doctor you would appreciate her giving the patient a large bolus of morphine or another sedative before discontinuing the ventilator, in order to prevent shortness of breath. If you have the slightest doubt about your loved one's comfort, tell your nurse, "I think he is uncomfortable. Would you please increase the pain medicine?"
- Understand that dying after withdrawal of life support can take between minutes to hours. Rarely, it can take days.
- After life support is discontinued, ask your nurse to silence alarms and, if you would like, to turn off the monitor display in the room. Ask if any tubes, lines, and restraints can be removed.
- Try not to be distracted by physical changes or changes on the monitors. Instead, concentrate on just being with your loved one.

AFTER DEATH

After your loved one dies, someone will come to the room to officially "pronounce" the patient dead. Each state has its own statutes about how this must be done. Usually, the person pronouncing death is a physician; usually, she will do a quick examination of the heart, lungs, pulses, and eyes.

Sometimes, pronouncing death occurs several minutes after the monitors have shown no heartbeat, and the family is well aware that the patient is dead. It can be confusing to have a physician then enter the room and examine the patient (the family can suddenly wonder, "My gosh, could my loved one actually still be *alive?*"). But pronouncing death is legally required, and often more ritualistic than diagnostic. For many families (and ICU caregivers), it serves the function of officially marking the end.

Most ICUs will be respectful of your desires to sit with your loved one after death until you are ready to go, even if that is for hours. You should not feel rushed. Similarly, you should not feel guilty about leaving the room when you are ready. Your loved one has already left. I think you will know the right time for you, whether it is immediately or hours later.

The family will need to make some arrangements and complete paperwork, with the help of hospital staff. You should take some time to yourself first, and if you haven't already done so, you may want to ask someone close to you to start managing the arrangements.

You or your helper should double-check whether your loved one has made a funeral plan, or whether he has left a "letter of instruction." The deceased will have sometimes named a "designated agent" to take care of his funeral arrangements. The hospital staff will help the family to contact a funeral home, if they choose to do so. In most states, the family is also permitted to collect the body and make funeral arrangements, if they prefer. Your relative's body will be cleaned, all remaining tubes and lines will be removed, and he may be taken to a hospital morgue until the funeral home or family members come to pick up the body. Very rarely – if the death was traumatic, unexpected, or suspicious – the body may first need to go to the coroner's office for inspection. If your loved one has previously made arrangements to donate his body to science (for example, to teach anatomy to medical students) there should be a preexisting contract with the medical institution. That contract will have a phone number to call to make arrangements for transportation.

What can you do?

There are many logistics to handle after death. If you are not in a state of mind to handle these, explicitly ask one of the people close to you to take charge of these arrangements.

AUTOPSY

ICU caretakers may ask whether you want an autopsy done before the body is released (and if they don't, you can request one). This is a very personal decision, and there is no right answer. Autopsies used to be fairly routine, because a minimum number were required to maintain the hospital's accreditation. That is no longer true, and autopsies are more infrequent. Moreover, insurers no longer pay for autopsies, so they may come at expense to the family. And of course, for many people, the idea of an autopsy on their loved one's body is upsetting.

Why might you want an autopsy? First, there is a societal benefit. Autopsies overall do provide an important function to the scientific understanding of disease, and to the ability of doctors and hospitals to get important feedback about their diagnoses and care. The fact that autopsies are now very rare is a blow to our understanding of disease and its treatment.

In terms of benefits to you and other family members, an autopsy might provide important information about what actually happened, and what caused your loved one's death. When the patient is alive, we do our best to deduce what is wrong through the pictures painted by lab results, other tests, and physical exams – but even excellent ICU doctors sometimes get the diagnosis wrong, and sometimes seriously wrong.[4] The question is: How important is it for you to be sure? Will it give you comfort to know the final diagnosis with certainty? Are you the kind of person who likes to have as much understanding as possible, even when the outcome is already determined? And if it turns out your loved one's caretakers *were* wrong, is that actually something you want to know, or is that something that might cause needless distress? When considering an autopsy, you should also be aware that in perhaps 1 in 20 cases, the autopsy does not provide conclusive evidence for the cause of death.[5]

Hospitals vary in whether and how much they charge for autopsies that they perform, so you may want to speak with a case manager before you decide (or ask a helper to do so). There is also the possibility of hiring a private autopsy, usually done at the funeral home or an outside facility, which typically costs $2,000–5,000.

* * * * * * *

Finally, let me close this chapter by saying how deeply sorry I am that you are losing, or have lost, your loved one. You should skip the next and last chapter of the book (except possibly, when you are ready, the last section, which deals with hospital bills). I hope you will read the conclusion of the book, however – it is the close of my long letter to you.

8

Surviving the ICU

You and your family member have come out on the other side of your ICU experience. The milestone of leaving the ICU is joyous – take a well-deserved moment to revel in that!

But afterward, gather your energies for the next phase. Although the most dangerous part is complete, the overall journey back to full health probably is not. Usually there are multiple residual issues that follow ICU patients and their families for weeks – or sometimes even years. This chapter of the book discusses some of these.

TRANSFER TO ELSEWHERE IN THE HOSPITAL

Most patients who leave the ICU are not discharged from the hospital immediately. Instead, they are transferred either to a general ward, or a step-down unit, which is a ward with more intensive monitoring capabilities (somewhere between a general ward and the ICU). On a general ward, you can expect that nurses have 4–7 patients, rather than 1–3 as in the ICU. There may no longer be continuous electronic monitoring of the patient's vital signs. There is still an attending physician – usually a specialist in hospital internal medicine called a "hospitalist" – but she may have many patients in many different areas of the hospital, and so may not always be close on hand. The transition is often disconcerting for families, who may have developed close relationships with ICU staff, and become accustomed to constant attention and monitoring in the ICU. Remember – the fact that your family member needs less attention and monitoring is a good sign!

But nervousness is not entirely without justification. The day or two immediately following transfer from the ICU is sometimes precarious. The patient is still fragile. For example, if he was previously on mechanical ventilation, he may still have low blood oxygen levels and thick sputum that is hard to cough up, making breathing difficult. There are different doctors and nurses on the new ward, and they don't yet know him well. Medications often change at the time of the transfer. During this transition, you can play an important role by bringing your new caregivers up to speed about your loved one, and by being at the bedside as much as possible to help alert caregivers to any changes you notice.

You can also play an important role in encouraging your relative's mobility, just as you may have done in the ICU. I've already explained the importance of mobility and exercise, in chapter 3. This is no less important now, and in fact probably increases in importance with every passing day. Moving around helps frail patients to avoid complications such as blood clots and pneumonia, and to regain muscle strength and balance. Now that your family member is well enough to be on the general ward, he is almost certainly well enough to do some exercise, and at least get out of bed to a chair for some time every day. Help to encourage mobility by questioning and reminding staff about it. Remember that your nurse will now have several other patients, and will find spending the time on mobility challenging. You can help the nurse by volunteering to help give support and supervision during exercise.

Part of mobility is respiratory exercise – taking deep breaths and coughing to expel sputum, and to prevent pneumonia. Just moving into a chair or taking a short walk helps a great deal with respiratory exercise. In addition, patients can use what is called an "incentive spirometer" several times throughout the day. The patient sucks on a mouthpiece to try to "lift" a ball as far as possible within a column – essentially forcing a prolonged, very deep breath.

What can you do?

- Ask for the name of your new "attending physician" or "hospitalist," and write it down. This is now the person with overall responsibility for your loved one, and the person to whom you should direct important questions. She will generally come to see your family member once a day, usually in the morning. If possible, try to be present then.

- During the first one or two days out of the ICU, spend as much time as you can at the bedside to be on the lookout for subtle changes in your loved one's condition. You will probably be more attuned to these than the new caregivers.
- Don't assume your new caregivers have a full understanding of all the details and events of the patient's ICU stay. Be as present as possible at the bedside to help fill in any holes in understanding.
- This is a very good time to make sure your physician knows what medications your relative was on at home, before the ICU admission. Some medications were probably stopped at the time of the admission, and at least some should probably now be restarted.
- If you have concerns about your loved one's breathing, ask your new attending physician whether the pulmonary (lung) doctors should follow along as consultants. Pulmonary physicians are often the same as the ICU doctors, so this may have the added benefit of keeping people who already know your loved one involved in his care. You could also ask your new attending physician whether she thinks it would be a good idea to order regular breathing treatments. This has the added advantage of bringing a respiratory therapist to the room at regular intervals, to help with respiratory monitoring and suctioning difficult-to-clear sputum.
- Ask your loved one's nurse every day about what the plans for mobility are, for example, getting out of bed to a chair. Volunteer to help by walking with your loved one, supervising him while sitting in a chair, or helping him with exercises.
- Ask your physician whether a physical therapy consult would be appropriate.
- Ask your physician whether your family member could have an incentive spirometer at the bedside, to use throughout the day.

DISCHARGE FROM THE HOSPITAL

Where ICU patients go after they leave the hospital depends very much on the nature of their critical illness. For example, at one extreme are patients who are essentially healthy but were in the ICU for intensive monitoring after surgery or another procedure; these patients may leave the hospital after a short stay and return quickly to their normal lives at home.

At the other extreme are patients who suffered severe manifestations of critical illness such as sepsis or acute respiratory distress syndrome (ARDS) and required days or even weeks of life support. These patients, as discussed in the section "Average prognosis for patients on prolonged life support" in chapter 6, are generally in for a long recovery, and remain at significant risk for recurrent problems that can send them back to the hospital. In this latter, sicker group of patients, only a minority go home after being discharged from the hospital. A fifth are discharged to an inpatient rehabilitation facility, where they undergo intensive therapy for several hours a day to try to improve their conditioning and physical functioning. About the same number go to a skilled nursing facility (SNF), where they will receive nursing care and general support. More than a third will go to a long-term acute care (LTAC) facility, which provides more intensive services and clinical care.[1] Some LTACs specialize in taking care of patients who still require a mechanical ventilator, but are otherwise considered stable. These facilities focus on ventilator weaning and respiratory care, physical rehabilitation, and nutrition. Often patients on mechanical ventilation stay in LTACs for more than a month (during which time most do successfully come off mechanical ventilation).

LTACs provide the advantage of expertise in ventilator weaning, and more attention to physical therapy, nutrition, counseling, and other issues important to full recovery. However, they are less equipped than an ICU to respond to complications and emergencies. It is important to recognize that part of the reason for the large increase in admissions to these facilities (threefold over one decade!) is changes in payment by insurers.[2] A subset of these transfers may not be appropriate. Patients should be transferred to ventilator weaning LTACs only when they are clinically stable and are expected to require additional prolonged mechanical ventilation. Particularly if the patient is nearly ready to come off the ventilator anyway, it may be safer to keep him in the ICU.

What can you do?

If your doctor is recommending that your loved one transfer to an LTAC while still needing a ventilator, ask for a full discussion of the risks and benefits. If your family member still has active medical problems or is reasonably likely to come off the ventilator within a week anyway, it may make more sense to avoid the risks of transfer and stay longer in the ICU. For example, you could start by saying something like, "I'm sure you understand that I'm nervous about being away from you and the other ICU specialists. Do you think he is completely stable at this point, and definitely won't get into trouble over there? Or would it be safer to keep him here?" You could also say, "I notice he's requiring less and less oxygen from the ventilator. Do you think there is a chance he could come off the ventilator in the next few days? If so, I'd really feel better if he could stay here during that time." And as always, it can be a game changer to ask what the doctor would recommend "if it were your family member."

POST-INTENSIVE CARE SYNDROME (PICS)

Post-intensive care syndrome, or PICS, refers to decreases in cognitive, psychiatric, and/or physical function that are often observed in patients after being in the ICU. There are many reasons for such decreases in function – a combination of the effects of the illness itself, pain and psychological trauma, loss of muscle strength with inactivity, and medications used in the ICU. The incidence and severity vary greatly with the nature of the critical illness – for example, a patient who is briefly in the ICU for routine monitoring after a procedure is unlikely to experience PICS. Factors that predispose to PICS include long ICU stays, the need for mechanical ventilation, severe disease such as ARDS or sepsis, and the use of certain medications such as paralytics, steroids, and sedatives. Overall, about half of ICU survivors will have at least one cognitive, psychiatric, or physical problem that persists for weeks, months, or even years after discharge.[3]

- *Cognitive impairment:* More than 1 in 4 ICU survivors have some decrease in their cognition, such as memory problems or difficulty with problem solving or concentration.[3] The rate is higher in patients with severe critical illness such as septic shock and ARDS. Cognitive impairments tend to improve over the first year after the ICU admission, but often persist to some extent for years.
- *Psychiatric impairment:* Many ICU survivors are left with psychological distress such as depression, anxiety, and post-traumatic stress disorder (PTSD).[4] PTSD symptoms may include nightmares, flashbacks, or obsessive thinking about the past ICU experience; hyperarousal with anxiety, restlessness, impulsivity, or aggression; and sometimes a dissociative or dream-like state. Three months after ICU admission, 16 percent of patients have PTSD, and 31 percent have depression.[5] It is estimated that almost half of patients have sleep disturbances.[6] As with cognitive

impairment, psychiatric problems may slowly improve, but often persist for years.

- *Physical impairment:* The most common physical impairment after an ICU stay is generalized weakness ("ICU weakness"), including weakness from specific types of muscle problems (critical illness myopathy) and nerve damage (critical illness polyneuropathy). Overall, at least 1 in 4 ICU patients have some degree of ICU weakness[7] – and as with cognitive and psychiatric impairment, the risk increases in very sick ICU patients, including those who required prolonged ventilation or had sepsis or ARDS. Use of paralytic medications and steroids are also risk factors. The impairment can range from mild weakness to near paralysis, causing significant dependence on caretakers. Physical limitation from ICU weakness may be exacerbated by deconditioning and malnutrition, as well as contractures (tightening) of the tendons, ligaments, and other tissues surrounding joints. Some patients, particularly if they were on mechanical ventilation, have problems with swallowing and speaking. The good news is that physical impairment after the ICU is likely to significantly improve over the first 2 years after the admission.

WHAT WILL YOUR ROLE BE WHEN YOUR LOVED ONE GOES HOME?

Whether because of PICS or other health problems, many patients require care and help with activities of daily living when they go home after an ICU admission. This requires a good deal of planning ahead of time.

The most important part of this planning is a realistic assessment of how much care and support the family or other people close to the patient can provide. For purposes of this discussion, I'll assume the primary caretaker among friends and family will be you, the reader. The amount of assistance needed varies greatly based on the nature of the critical illness. Most patients who had long ICU stays and mechanical ventilation (for example, because of septic shock or ARDS) have at least some dependence on caregivers even one year after discharge, and half of these will be nearly completely dependent.[1] For ICU patients who received more than 2 days of mechanical ventilation before going home, family caregivers spend an average of more than five hours per day giving care for at least the first half year (that's more than a half-time job). The majority of these caregivers are unemployed; more than 10 percent stop work specifically to care for their loved one.[8] Of those caregivers who continue working, almost a third have to reduce their work hours.[9]

For some family members, this kind of investment of personal time is just not possible – economically, or in terms of balancing other responsibilities. Right now you probably are so focused on your loved one, and so grateful for his survival, that you feel ready for personal sacrifice. But this is a marathon, not a sprint, and you need to make a realistic assessment of what is sustainable in the long run.

DISCHARGE PLANNING

Once you have a clear understanding of the amount of caregiving you can provide, you are ready to realistically plan discharge to home. The hospital (or other facility) has a "discharge planner" or "discharge case manager" to help. Ask to speak with this person well before you think your loved one is ready to go home, as there may be a lot of arrangements to make. Asking, "Will there be a discharge planner assigned to us, and might I start talking to them today?" will usually get you pointed in the right direction.

Speak frankly to the discharge planner about the role you will be able to play after your loved one goes home, and the number of hours per day you can realistically spend helping. This will affect the timing of discharge, as well as the amount of home services (for example, home nursing care) you receive. Medicare and other insurers will pay for some home nursing services if they are determined "medically necessary" by a physician. Similarly, you should work with the discharge planner to arrange for any medical equipment you will need at home. "Durable medical equipment" will also be covered by most insurers – if you, the discharge planner, and your doctors jump through the right hoops. This includes equipment like wheelchairs, walkers, hospital beds, bedside toilets, blood sugar monitors, oxygen and respiratory equipment, and patient lifts. A doctor will need to write a prescription for the equipment to be sent to a Home Medical Equipment (HME) provider, as well as a note documenting that the equipment is "medically necessary" and documenting specific criteria to be eligible for payment.

Get to work arranging these services and equipment as early as possible, to take advantage of the ready availability of the hospital doctors and case managers. Once your relative is discharged, they will disappear like Cinderella's coach, and you will probably have to pursue any loose ends with your loved one's primary care physician. Ask your discharge planner to give you copies of what prescriptions and documentation were sent to which Home Medical Equipment (HME) provider, in case you need to follow up on any equipment that doesn't materialize. If you are told that your insurance doesn't cover an item, it isn't necessarily true – you can try calling the HME provider to ask what is needed to qualify, and go back to the discharge planner or doctor for the necessary documentation.

In addition, you may want to prepare your home with equipment not typically covered by insurance, like grab bars in the bathroom, emergency communicators, exercise equipment, or stair lifts.

Finally, make sure your loved one has any follow-up appointments (for doctors' visits, tests, or therapy) definitely scheduled *before* you leave the hospital. If hospital staff give you a list of suggested appointments (rather than schedule them for you), start making the calls to get them scheduled before your family member is discharged. If you are having trouble getting the appointments scheduled in an appropriate time frame, you can enlist the help of doctors and case managers while you are still in the hospital. If your loved one has not had a primary care physician previously, this is the time to establish care with one.

POST-ICU RESOURCES AND CARE

The Society for Critical Care Medicine (SCCM) has an online initiative called "Thrive," designed to support patients and their families after an ICU admission.[10] Thrive provides information about PICS and about various resources, including connections to online support groups.

Your loved one may have chronic medical conditions or specific new problems that require medical follow-up after discharge. In addition, in the likely event that he has manifestations of PICS, some follow-up will be necessary. I would suggest that any person who has had an ICU stay should be seen by their primary care physician as soon as possible after discharge, and, if he has PICS, at least every month or two, to begin with. Some health care organizations provide "PICS clinics" or "after-ICU clinics," designed specifically to take care of patients after an ICU admission. The SCCM Thrive website provides a partial list of these clinics throughout the United States. Check this list, and also check with your local health care organizations to see if you can find a nearby after-ICU clinic.

If you cannot identify a local after-ICU clinic, your primary care physician will take charge of your loved one's after-ICU care. In addition to taking care of underlying medical conditions, she may need to coordinate support in the three main areas of PICS: cognitive, mental health, and physical function. The following support might be needed:

- *Psychiatrist or psychologist:* Your loved one has just lived through a traumatic experience, and is quite possibly wrestling with the new reality of dependence on others, ongoing pain or other symptoms, and interruption of employment. There is no shame in seeking counseling or therapy to help support someone after this kind of profound life change.
- *Physiatrist and/or physical therapist:* Your relative quite likely has weakness or other physical impairments, and would benefit from a supervised program of rehabilitation.
- *Occupational therapist:* An occupational therapist works with patients to help them regain independence in activities of daily living such as feeding, dressing, bathing, and grooming.
- *Speech therapist:* This person specializes in the mechanics of speaking and swallowing, and may be useful particularly if your relative has been on mechanical ventilation or has had a neurological injury that affects these mechanics. A speech therapist can work with your loved one on pronunciation and fluency. He or she can evaluate swallowing function, and make recommendations for how to eat safely, minimizing the risk of inhaling food. (See the section "Long-term feeding tubes" in chapter 4 for a discussion of swallowing tests – remember that these should ideally be performed after removal of temporary feeding tubes and tracheostomy tubes, to optimize swallowing ability.)

What can you do to get ready for discharge?

- Make a realistic assessment of the time you and other family will be able to spend taking care of your family member when he is home.
- Ask to speak with a discharge planner early.
- Work with the discharge planner to arrange for any durable medical equipment (DME) you will need at home. He or she can help to make sure that your insurance has the appropriate documentation of necessity from the doctor, so that the charge is covered. Also think about what other non-covered equipment might make things easier at home.
- Ask to have copies of any prescriptions/documentation sent to home medical equipment (HME) providers, so that you can follow up on any missing equipment.
- Investigate whether there are any local "after-ICU" or "PICS" clinics.
- Schedule an appointment as soon as possible with your family member's primary care physician (if he doesn't have one, this is the time

to establish care). Among other things, if your loved one has PICS, his primary care physician will be important to coordinating the necessary care.

- Ask your hospital doctor what other follow-up appointments will be needed, and try to get these scheduled before you leave the hospital, enlisting the help of hospital staff if necessary. They can often help get more timely appointments, if you are having trouble.

EXERCISE AFTER THE ICU

By now you probably have realized that I'm a strong believer in keeping patients moving and exercising as much as possible during their critical illness and hospitalization. This is just as important for patients after they go home.[11] If elderly and frail people stop moving, they become vulnerable to mishaps like falls, blood clots, and pneumonia. This can be a vicious cycle: frailty and immobility lead to complications, which lead to more frailty and immobility, which lead to further complications, and so forth. Breaking out of this downward spiral takes real determination, and your support for your relative can help a lot.

If your relative has certain problems with heart or lungs, health insurance may cover outpatient cardiac or pulmonary rehabilitation. This is a program of several months of supervised exercise and health education, usually meeting 2–3 times per week, prescribed by a physician. For certain conditions like chronic obstructive pulmonary disease (COPD) – smoker's lung disease – pulmonary rehabilitation has been shown to have powerful effects: improved quality of life, higher exercise tolerance, fewer and shorter hospitalizations, and even decreased mortality. Even if your relative is not eligible for intensive cardiac or pulmonary rehabilitation, your relative's physician may be able to prescribe some physical therapy. For some people, it may be an option to hire a personal trainer to help.

Expert supervision is a great thing, but there is a lot your loved one can do on his own, with your support. Exactly *how* he exercises is less important than that he *does* exercise. The trick is to be regular and intentional, and keep to a schedule – absolutely no excuses! Scheduling exercise with a friend or a trainer can help to maintain motivation. Set aside two inviolate periods of time every day to exercise, and every day make a point to include stretches, muscle strength building, and cardiopulmonary exercise (which increases breathing and heart rate). Keep a journal of what is done and for how long, in order to track progress. It is not important to make rapid progress – just to make at least a little progress every week. Exercise should be hard enough to be somewhat unpleasant (without being painful). It should get your loved one's heart rate up, make him breathe harder, and possibly sweat. Review the exercise plan with his doctor, and discuss any medical limitations – for example, a patient with heart disease should not exercise if he is having chest pain.

PAYING FOR IT ALL

The United States, alone among all advanced countries, charges patients for each episode of illness, as though care were an optional market commodity. The more serious the illness, the higher the charges. Other countries have publicly funded universal health care without charging by illness. In the United States, even those who are insured face large out-of-pocket costs. Because of the callousness of this market-based system, patients in the ICU and their families are hit twice – first, by a serious illness, and second by having to pay for it as if it were a privilege. The result is that if you live in the United States, your loved one's stay in the ICU will probably leave your family with a heavy financial burden – as if you didn't have enough on your plate already.

The charges for an ICU admission vary widely depending on how long and complicated it is. For patients who have severe critical illness (for example, those with ARDS, shock, and/or prolonged mechanical ventilation), total charges of hospitalization average well over $200,000, and total one-year charges (including follow-up care and subsequent hospitalizations) average well over $300,000.[1] At the same time, both the patient and family caretakers are likely to experience significant decreases in employment and income after an ICU stay.[10, 12, 13] Almost half of family members report suffering serious financial stress 3 months after an ICU admission.[14]

The challenges posed by these circumstances are reflected in the fact that, even after the Affordable Care Act expanded insurance coverage, two-thirds of bankruptcies filed in the United States are attributed to medical bills,[15] and medical bills represent over half of overdue credit card debt.[16] One-third of GoFundMe campaigns are for medical bills.[17]

What can you do to help tackle this financial burden? The first thing to do is to recognize that financial difficulties stemming from an ICU stay are common, not your fault, and not shameful. The shame lies in a health care system that leaves people who are unlucky enough to get sick to the wolves. Residents of other advanced countries do not experience this kind of heartlessness.

Now . . . what can you do on a practical level?

It is common for medical bills to contain errors and overcharges – which can be corrected. In addition, it's sometimes possible to negotiate discounts, or at least more feasible payment plans. Finally, it's sometimes possible to appeal insurance coverage decisions. In this case as in many others, the saying "the squeaky wheel gets the grease" is true. But being a squeaky wheel takes time and patience, and you are likely now occupied by helping to coordinate or provide care for your loved one. Make the decision whether it is worth it to you to invest the considerable effort needed to dispute or renegotiate bills and insurance coverage. Consider asking family and friends for help – either directly, or by spending time occasionally caring for your relative so that you can have time to concentrate on dealing with medical bills. If you are able to do so, consider hiring a medical billing advocate to do the legwork – they generally will charge from 20–30 percent of the savings they achieve on your behalf (and they often do achieve significant savings).

If you are handling the bills – and particularly if you are considering contesting the price tag – get organized right away. In general, you have 90 days to dispute medical bills. (Once you know what charges you plan to dispute, you can ask the hospital billing department if they will hold off on sending the bill to collection agencies to give you some additional time.) Be meticulous. Keep every relevant bill and document that you receive. Make a record of the date, time, and content of every phone conversation. Send any mail as certified mail with a return receipt, so that you can document receipt of the communication if necessary.

What can you do?

These are the basic steps to pursue:

- Request a line-item bill from the hospital billing department. (The bill you are initially sent will likely provide an overall summary of charges, but you want the details.) Charges are often listed by current procedural code (CPT), a five-digit number. If not defined on the bill, it's easy to find the meaning of CPT codes with an online search. Review the bill for unexpected charges or amounts. Sometimes billing mistakes take the form of a single digit change in CPT code, which can mean thousands of dollars.
- In addition to charges that stand out as wrong or too high, look for discrepancies with "explanation of benefits" documents from your insurance company. The amounts listed on these documents for

what you owe your provider should correspond to amounts on your bills from the hospital.

- For charges that seem excessive, find out what other hospitals are charging for the same CPT, for example through websites such as *Clear Health Costs*, *Healthcare Blue Book*, and *Fair Health*.
- Call the billing department to contest specific charges, or to request an audit of the bill for accuracy. You can also try to renegotiate payment. People are sometimes surprised at what they can achieve simply by asking. Occasionally, billing departments will provide a discount if you are able to pay the full bill immediately. Or they may be able to provide an extended payment plan if you need more time. You may be eligible for hospital financial assistance. If you are not making any headway, ask to speak with a supervisor, and then, if necessary, that person's supervisor. Often, the people on the front lines are not empowered to offer discounts, while more senior people are.
- Consider contacting the hospital's patient advocate. These people work for the hospital, but usually take their job representing patients very seriously. They may help to renegotiate charges and payment plans with the billing department, and sometimes they themselves are empowered to offer discounts. They are also good at finding other community resources to help.
- If you think the hospital has made an error and wrongly charged you, but you aren't making headway with the billing department, consider filing an appeal with your insurance company. Your insurance company is also interested in not being overcharged by the hospital, and may become a powerful ally.
- If you think your insurance company has wrongly denied coverage, consider filing an appeal with your state's insurance commissioner.

Conclusion

How Will You Be after the ICU?

What does life hold for you after the ICU? How will you have changed, and how will you look back on the experience? In some respects, you and I now have something in common – an intense immersion in a world that few others know. It is powerful, but also isolating. Not many people will be able to understand fully what you have gone through.

Your experience has no doubt been difficult and distressing, at least at times. In fact, family members of ICU patients are almost as likely as the patients themselves to experience residual psychological effects, including anxiety and depression. More than 1 in 10 family members will have symptoms of post-traumatic stress disorder (PTSD).[1] This is particularly true of people whose family members have died in the ICU, and even more so for people who have been involved in making the decision to withdraw life support for a loved one.[2] It seems unfair to me that this act of courage and love should leave people so devastated, even beyond the fact that someone they love has died.

Part of what makes the ICU experience so traumatic for family members is lack of information, and perceived lack of control. My great hope is that this book gave you information you needed not to be overwhelmed by the ICU environment, to be a capable advocate for your loved one, and to have a sense of agency and understanding of your own central role.

Now that your time in the ICU is over, I have two suggestions – really, requests. First, please don't look back and second guess your actions and decisions. You operated as well as you possibly could under extremely trying and stressful circumstances. You probably made some hard decisions: most of the time, such decisions are hard because no one answer is clearly right, and you are choosing among incredibly difficult alternatives. Be forgiving and understanding toward yourself, as I expect your loved one is or would be.

Second, find someone to talk with about your experiences. You might consider seeing a psychologist or psychiatrist. You have been through a very difficult experience, and the rest of your life has perhaps been upended – there is no shame in seeking help. Alternatively, consider joining a family support group, where you can talk to people who will understand what you went through (the Society of Critical Care Medicine initiative "Thrive" includes information about family support groups on its website).[3] You have given plenty of time to your family member – now, make some time for yourself.

Although the stressors of the ICU experience are obvious and their negative effects on family members well documented, I think there is another side of the story that isn't as well told – the glorious things that come from people at the moments when we are most tested. I suspect that you were stronger, smarter, braver, and more loving than you have ever been. Perhaps you know that. Perhaps you learned things about yourself, your loved one, and your relationship that you had not known. I said in the preface to this book that the great privilege of the ICU is being allowed to be part of the heart of what matters. Perhaps now you see that the heart of what mattered was you.

Appendix

Use the table on the next page as a guide to questions for nurses and doctors that may help to prevent typical complications of ICU care.

SUPPORTING THE PREVENTION OF COMPLICATIONS: DAILY QUESTIONS FOR THE ICU TEAM

Date: _____ Name of ICU Nurse: _____
Name of ICU Doctor: _____

QUESTIONS	NOTES
Are there any lines or tubes that can come out today? (If not, what specifically are the indications to continue?) • Endotracheal tube • Central line or PICC • Urinary catheter • Chest tube	
If on a ventilator: Did the patient have a spontaneous breathing trial this morning? (If not, what were the specific contraindications?)	
If on sedative medications: • Did the patient have a sedation vacation this morning? (If not, what were the specific contraindications?) Did he wake up, and how was he? • *If too sleepy to sustain eye-contact:* Would it be possible to lighten sedation at all?	
What are the plans for mobility today? Examples: • Regular turning • Sitting upright (how long?) • Passive range of motion • Active range of motion • Out of bed to a chair (how long?) • Standing or walking	
Could I help you today with: • Supervising patient during lighter sedation • Assisting with mobility/exercise • Swabbing patient's mouth	
Medications: • Have any new medications been started? If so, what are the possible side effects? • Is the patient on gastric acid suppression? If so, could sucralfate be used instead? • Are there any antibiotics that could be stopped or changed to narrower spectrum antibiotics today?	
Nutrition: • Is the patient receiving tube feeds? If so, is he "at goal"?	

Notes

INTRODUCTION

1. "Critical Care Statistics," SCCM.org, Society of Critical Care Medicine, accessed January 24, 2021, https://www.sccm.org/Communications/Critical-Care-Statistics.

2. Derek C. Angus et al., "Use of intensive care at the end of life in the United States: An epidemiologic study," *Critical Care Medicine* 32, no. 3 (March 2004): 638.

CHAPTER 1

1. Andres Esteban et al., "Characteristics and outcomes in adult patients receiving mechanical ventilation: A 28-day international study," *Journal of the American Medical Association* 287, no. 3 (January 2002): 345.

2. Lars W. Andersen et al., "In-hospital cardiac arrest: A review," *Journal of the American Medical Association* 321, no. 12 (March 2019): 1202.

3. Paul S. Chan et al., "Long-term outcomes in elderly survivors of in-hospital cardiac arrest," *New England Journal of Medicine* 368, no. 11 (March 2013): 1023.

4. Patricia Jabre et al., "Family presence during cardiopulmonary resuscitation," *New England Journal of Medicine* 368, no. 11 (March 2013): 1008.

CHAPTER 2

1. Flavio Lopes Ferreira et al., "Serial evaluation of the SOFA score to predict outcome in critically ill patients," *Journal of the American Medical Association* 286, no. 14 (October 2001): 1754.

2. Timothy D. Girard et al., "Efficacy and safety of a paired sedation and ventilator weaning protocol for mechanically ventilated patients in intensive care (Awakening and Breathing Controlled trial): A randomized controlled trial," *The Lancet* 371, no. 9607 (January 2008): 126.

3. Theodore J. Iwashyna et al., "Uncharted paths: Hospital networks in critical care," *Chest* 135, no. 3 (March 2009): 828.

4. Jeffrey M. Singh et al., "Critical events during land-based interfacility transport," *Annals of Emergency Medicine* 64, no. 1 (July 2014): 9.

5. Yasser Sakr et al., "The impact of hospital and ICU organizational factors on outcome in critically ill patients: Results from the extended prevalence of infection in intensive care study," *Critical Care Medicine* 43, no. 3 (March 2015): 519.

6. Matlin Gilman et al., "Safety-net hospitals more likely than other hospitals to fare poorly under Medicare's Value-Based Purchasing," *Health Affairs* 34, no. 3 (March 2015): 398.

CHAPTER 3

1. Prasoon Jain et al., "Overuse of the indwelling urinary tract catheter in hospitalized medical patients," *Archives of Internal Medicine* 155, no. 13 (July 1995): 1425.

2. J. Thomas Lamont et al., "Clostridioides Difficile infection in adults: Epidemiology, microbiology, and pathophysiology," UpToDate, accessed February 20, 2021. https://www.uptodate.com/contents/clostridioides-formerly-clostridium-difficile -infection-in-adults-epidemiology-microbiology-and-pathophysiology.

3. Society for Hospital Epidemiology of America et al., "Consensus paper on the surveillance of surgical wound infections," *Infection Control and Hospital Epidemiology* 13, no. 10 (October 1992): 599.

4. Rodrigo Cavallazzi et al., "Delirium in the ICU: An overview," *Annals of Intensive Care* 2, no. 1 (December 2012): 49.

5. Theodoros Ladopoulos, "Gastrointestinal dysmotility in critically ill patients," *Annals of Gastroenterology* 31, no. 3 (March 2018): 1.

6. Lucian L. Leape et al., "The nature of adverse events in hospitalized patients: Results of the Harvard Medical Practice Study II," *New England Journal of Medicine* 324, no. 6 (February 1991): 377.

7. Bernard De Jonghe et al., "Paresis acquired in the intensive care unit: A prospective multicenter study," *Journal of the American Medical Association* 288, no. 22 (December 2002): 2859.

CHAPTER 4

1. Calvin A. Brown et al., "Rapid sequence intubation for adults outside the operating room," UpToDate, accessed February 17, 2021, https://www.uptodate.com/contents/rapid-sequence-intubation-for-adults-outside-the-operating-room.

2. Michael P. Young et al., "Overview of complications of central venous catheters and their prevention," UpToDate, accessed February 17, 2021, https://www.upto date.com/contents/overview-of-complications-of-central-venous-catheters-and-their -prevention.

3. Arthur C. Theodore et al., "Intra-arterial catheterization for invasive monitoring: Indications, insertion techniques, and interpretation," UpToDate, accessed February 17, 2021, https://www.uptodate.com/contents/intra-arterial-catheterization-for -invasive-monitoring-indications-insertion-techniques-and-interpretation.

4. Jeffrey L. Carson et al., "Indications and hemoglobin thresholds for red blood cell transfusion in the adult," UpToDate, accessed February 17, 2021, https://www .uptodate.com/contents/indications-and-hemoglobin-thresholds-for-red-blood-cell -transfusion-in-the-adult.

5. Arthur J. Silvergleid, "Immunologic transfusion reactions," UpToDate, accessed February 17, 2021, https://www.uptodate.com/contents/immunologic-transfusion -reactions.

6. John E. Heffner et al., "Ultrasound-guided thoracentesis," UpToDate, accessed February 17, 2021, https://www.uptodate.com/contents/ultrasound-guided-thoracen tesis.

7. John T. Huggins et al., "Large volume (therapeutic) thoracentesis: Procedure and complications," UpToDate, accessed February 17, 2021, https://www.uptodate .com/contents/large-volume-therapeutic-thoracentesis-procedure-and-complications.

8. John T. Huggins et al., "Thoracostomy tubes and catheters: Placement techniques and complications," UpToDate, accessed February 17, 2021, https://www.uptodate.com/contents/thoracostomy-tubes-and-catheters-placement-techniques-and-complications.

9. Gerald L. Weinhouse, "Pulmonary artery catheterization: Indications, contra-indications, and complications in adults," UpToDate, accessed February 17, 2021, https://www.uptodate.com/contents/pulmonary-artery-catheterization-indications -contraindications-and-complications-in-adults.

10. Thomas J. Kearney et al., "Pulmonary artery rupture associated with the Swan-Ganz catheter," *Chest* 108, no. 5 (November 1995): 1349.

11. Shaheen Islam, "Flexible bronchoscopy in adults: Preparation, procedural technique, and complications," UpToDate, accessed February 17, 2021, https:// www.uptodate.com/contents/flexible-bronchoscopy-in-adults-preparation-procedural -technique-and-complications.

12. Stephen E. Silvis et al., "Endoscopic complications: Results of the 1974 American Society for Gastrointestinal Endoscopy Survey," *Journal of the American Medical Association* 235, no. 9 (March 1976): 928.

13. Askar Chukmaitov et al., "Association of polypectomy techniques, endoscopist volume, and facility type with colonoscopy complications," *Gastrointestinal Endoscopy* 77, no. 3 (March 2013): 436.

14. Jonathan Cohen et al., "Overview of upper gastrointestinal endoscopy (esophagogastroduodenoscopy)," UpToDate, accessed February 17, 2021, https://www.uptodate.com/contents/overview-of-upper-gastrointestinal-endoscopy-esophago gastroduodenoscopy.

15. Linda Lee et al., "Overview of colonoscopy in adults," UpToDate, accessed February 17, 2021, https://www.uptodate.com/contents/overview-of-colonoscopy-in-adults.

16. Bruce A. Runyon, "Diagnostic and therapeutic abdominal paracentesis," UpToDate, accessed February 17, 2021, https://www.uptodate.com/contents/diagnostic-and-therapeutic-abdominal-paracentesis.

17. Peter F. Fedullo et al., "Placement of vena cava filters and their complications," UpToDate, accessed February 17, 2021, https://www.uptodate.com/contents/placement-of-vena-cava-filters-and-their-complications.

18. Eun Cho et al., "Failed inferior vena cava filter retrieval by conventional method: Analysis of its causes and retrieval of it by modified double-loop technique," *Phlebology* 30, no. 8 (September 2015): 549.

19. Joseph P. Carrozza, "Complications of diagnostic cardiac catheterization," UpToDate, accessed February 2021, https://www.uptodate.com/contents/complications-of-diagnostic-cardiac-catheterization.

20. H. Vernon Anderson et al., "A contemporary overview of percutaneous coronary interventions: The American College of Cardiology-National Cardiovascular Data Registry (ACC-NCDR)," *Journal of the American College of Cardiology* 39, no. 7 (April 2002): 1096.

21. Joseph P. Carrozza, "Complications of diagnostic cardiac catheterization," UpToDate, accessed February 2021, https://www.uptodate.com/contents/complica tions-of-diagnostic-cardiac-catheterization; and Joseph P. Carrozza, "Periprocedural complications of percutaneous coronary intervention," UpToDate, accessed February 17, 2021, https://www.uptodate.com/contents/periprocedural-complications-of -percutaneous-coronary-intervention.

22. Sung-Min Cho et al., "Radiographic and clinical brain infarcts in cardiac and diagnostic procedures," *Stroke* 48, no. 10 (September 2017): 2753.

23. F. V. Y. Tjong et al., "A comprehensive scoping review on transvenous tempo-rary pacing therapy," *Netherlands Heart Journal* 27 (August 2019): 462.

24. Edward R. Smith et al., "Evaluation and management of elevated intracranial pressure in adults," UpToDate, accessed February 17, 2021, https://www.uptodate.com/contents/evaluation-and-management-of-elevated-intracranial-pressure-in-adults.

25. Jean L. Holley, "Acute complications during hemodialysis," UpToDate, accessed February 17, 2021, https://www.uptodate.com/contents/acute-complications-during -hemodialysis.

26. James J. Ferguson et al., "The current practice of intra-aortic balloon counter-pulsation: Results from the Benchmark Registry," *Journal of the American College of Cardiology* 38, no. 5 (November 2001): 1456.

27. Roger J. Laham et al., "Intraaortic balloon pump counterpulsation," UpToDate, accessed February 17, 2021, https://www.uptodate.com/contents/intraaortic-balloon-pump-counterpulsation.

28. Robert Bartlett, "Extracorporeal membrane oxygenation (ECMO) in adults," UpToDate, accessed February 17, 2021, https://www.uptodate.com/contents/extracorporeal-membrane-oxygenation-ecmo-in-adults.

29. Jason T. Chapman et al., "CNS complications in adult patients treated with extracorporeal membrane oxygenation," *Critical Care Medicine* 49, no. 2 (February 2021): 282.

30. Farrah J. Mateen et al., "Neurological injury in adults treated with extracorporeal membrane oxygenation," *Archives of Neurology* 68, no. 12 (December 2011): 1543.

31. Robert C. Hyzy et al., "Overview of tracheostomy," UpToDate, accessed February 17, 2021, https://www.uptodate.com/contents/overview-of-tracheostomy.

32. Paul Scalise et al., "The incidence of tracheoarterial fistula in patients with chronic tracheostomy tubes: A retrospective study of 544 patients in a long-term care facility," *Chest* 128, no. 6 (December 2005): 3906.

33. Anica C. Law et al., "Gastrostomy tube use in the critically ill, 1994–2014," *Annals of the American Thoracic Society* 16, no. 6 (June 2019): 724.

34. Mark H. DeLegge, "Gastrostomy tubes: Complications and their management," UpToDate, accessed February 17, 2021, https://www.uptodate.com/contents/gastrostomy-tubes-complications-and-their-management.

35. Y. Zopf et al., "Local infection after placement of percutaneous endoscopic gastrostomy tubes: A prospective study evaluating risk factors," *Canadian Journal of Gastroenterology* 22, no. 12 (December 2008): 987.

CHAPTER 5

1. Lida P. Hariri et al., "Lung histopathology in coronavirus disease 2019 as compared with severe acute respiratory syndrome and H1N1 influenza: A systematic review," *Chest* 159, no. 1 (January 2021): 73.

2. Daniel E. Leisman et al., "Cytokine elevation in severe and critical COVID-19: A rapid systematic review, meta-analysis, and comparison with other inflammatory syndromes," *Lancet Respiratory Medicine* 8, no. 12 (December 2020): 1233.

3. Haziq Siddiqi, "To suffer alone: Hospital visitation policies during COVID-19," *Journal of Hospital Medicine* 15, no. 11 (November 2020): 694–695.

4. "State operations manual, Appendix A: Survey protocol, regulations and interpretive guidelines for hospitals," Centers for Medicare and Medicaid Services, CMS.gov, accessed February 9, 2021, https://www.cms.gov/regulations-and-guidance/guidance/transmittals/downloads/r75soma.pdf.

5. "Hospital visitation: Phase II visitation for patients who are Covid-19 negative," Centers for Medicare and Medicaid Services, CMS.gov, accessed February 9, 2021,

https://www.cms.gov/files/document/covid-hospital-visitation-phase-ii-visitation-covid-negative-patients.pdf.

6. "Operational considerations for adapting a contact tracing program to respond to the COVID-19 pandemic," Centers for Disease Control and Prevention, CDC.gov, accessed February 9, 2021, https://www.cdc.gov/coronavirus/2019-ncov/global-covid-19/operational-considerations-contact-tracing.html#.

7. Atul Malhotra et al., "Prone ventilation for adult patients with acute respiratory distress syndrome," UpToDate, accessed February 9, 2021, https://www.upto date.com/contents/prone-ventilation-for-adult-patients-with-acute-respiratory-distress-syndrome.

8. Carlos Ferrando et al., "Clinical features, ventilatory management, and outcome of ARDS caused by COVID-19 are similar to other causes of ARDS," *Intensive Care Medicine* 46, no. 12 (December 2020): 2200.

9. Eddy Fan et al., "COVID-19 associated acute respiratory distress syndrome: Is a different approach to management warranted?" *Lancet Respiratory Medicine* 8, no. 8 (August 2020): 816.

10. Anne-Fleur Haudebourg et al., "Respiratory mechanics of COVID-19-versus non-COVID-19-associated respiratory distress syndrome," *American Journal of Respiratory and Critical Care Medicine* 202, no. 2 (July 2020): 287.

11. "Trials halt full-dose clot prophylaxix for severe COVID-19," Medpage Today, accessed February 14, 2021, https://www.medpagetoday.com/infectiousdisease/covid19/90351.

12. Peter Hornby et al., "Dexamethasone in hospitalized patients with Covid-19: Preliminary report," *New England Journal of Medicine*, published ahead of print, July 17, 2020, https://doi.org/10.1056/NEJMoa2021436.

13. John H. Beigel et al., "Remdesivir for the treatment of Covid-19: Final report," *New England Journal of Medicine* 383, no. 19 (November 2020): 1813.

14. Reed Siemieniuk et al., "Drug treatments for covid-19: Living systematic review and network meta-analysis," *British Medical Journal*, published ahead of print, July 30, 2020. https://doi.org/10.1136/bmj.m2980.

15. Joseph M. Unger et al., "The scientific impact of positive and negative phase III cancer clinical trials," *Journal of the American Medical Association Oncology* 2, no. 7 (July 2016): 875.

16. Conor Hale, "New MIT Study Puts Clinical Research Success Rate at 14 Percent," CenterWatch, accessed February 16, 2021, https://www.centerwatch.com/articles/12702-new-mit-study-puts-clinical-research-success-rate-at-14-percent.

17. Adam Cuker et al., "Coronavirus disease 2019 (COVID-19): Hypercoagulability," UpToDate, accessed February 14, 2021, https://www.uptodate.com/contents/coronavirus-disease-2019-covid-19-hypercoagulability.

18. Gideon Meyerowitz-Katz et al., "A systematic review and meta-analysis of published research data on COVID-19 infection fatality rates," *International Journal of Infectious Diseases*, published ahead of print, September 29, 2020, https://doi.org/10.1016/j.ijid.2020.09.1464.

19. George L. Anesi, "Coronavirus disease 2019 (COVID-19): Critical care and airway management issues," UpToDate, accessed February 14, 2021, https://www .uptodate.com/contents/coronavirus-disease-2019-covid-19-critical-care-and-airway -management-issues.

20. Farhaan S. Vahidy et al., "Characteristics and outcomes of COVID-19 patients during initial peak and resurgence in the Houston metropolitan area," *Journal of the American Medical Association* 324, no. 10 (September 2020): 998.

21. Sara C. Auld et al., "ICU and ventilator mortality among critically ill adults with coronavirus disease 2019," *Critical Care Medicine* 48, no. 9 (September 2020): e800.

22. Katherine Mackey et al., "Racial and ethnic disparities in COVID-19-related infections, hospitalizations, and deaths," *Annals of Internal Medicine*, published ahead of print, December 1, 2020, https://doi.org/10.7326/M20-6306.

23. Matthew J. Cummings et al., "Epidemiology, clinical course, and outcomes of critically ill adults with COVID-19 in New York City: A prospective cohort study," *Lancet* 395, no. 10239 (June 2020): 1763.

24. Mark D. Siegel et al., "Acute respiratory distress syndrome: Prognosis and outcomes in adults," UpToDate, accessed February 15, 2021, https://www.uptodate .com/contents/acute-respiratory-distress-syndrome-prognosis-and-outcomes-in-adults.

25. Mark E. Mikkelsen et al., "The adult respiratory distress syndrome cognitive outcomes study: Long-term neuropsychological function in survivors of acute lung injury," *American Journal of Respiratory and Critical Care Medicine* 185, no. 12 (June 2012): 1307.

26. Chaolin Huang et al., "6-month consequences of COVID-19 in patients discharged from hospital: A cohort study," *Lancet* 397, no. 10270 (January 2021): 220.

27. Margaret S. Herridge et al., "Functional disability 5 years after acute respiratory distress syndrome," *New England Journal of Medicine* 364, no. 14 (April 2011): 1293.

28. Oscar J. Bienvenu et al., "Depressive symptoms and impaired physical function after acute lung injury: A 2-year longitudinal study," *American Journal of Respiratory and Critical Care Medicine* 185, no. 5 (March 2012): 517.

CHAPTER 6

1. Vivek K. Moitra et al., "Relationship between ICU length of stay and long-term mortality for elderly ICU survivors," *Critical Care Medicine* 44, no. 4 (April 2016): 655.

2. A. R. Manara et al., "Reasons for withdrawing treatment in patients receiving intensive care," *Anaesthesia* 53, no. 6 (June 1998): 523.

3. Elie Azoulay et al., "Risk of post-traumatic stress symptoms in family members of intensive care patients," *American Journal of Respiratory and Critical Care Medicine* 171, no. 9 (May 2005): 987.

4. Cynthia J. Gries et al., "Predictors of symptoms of posttraumatic stress and depression in family members after patient death in the ICU," *Chest* 137, no. 2 (February 2010): 283.

5. Mark Unroe et al., "One-year trajectories of care and resource utilization for recipients of prolonged mechanical ventilation: A cohort study," *Annals of Internal Medicine* 153, no. 3 (August 2010): 171.

6. MeiLan King Han, "Management and prognosis of patients requiring prolonged mechanical ventilation," UpToDate, accessed February 15, 2021, https://www.uptodate.com/contents/management-and-prognosis-of-patients-requiring-prolonged-mechanical-ventilation.

7. Mark D. Siegel et al., "Acute respiratory distress syndrome: Prognosis and outcomes in adults," UpToDate, accessed February 15, 2021, https://www.uptodate.com/contents/acute-respiratory-distress-syndrome-prognosis-and-outcomes-in-adults.

8. Alain Combes et al., "Morbidity, mortality, and quality-of-life outcomes of patients requiring > or = 14 days of mechanical ventilation," *Critical Care Medicine* 31, no. 5 (May 2003): 1373.

9. Christopher E. Cox et al., "Expectations and outcomes of prolonged mechanical ventilation," *Critical Care Medicine* 37, no. 11 (November 2009): 2888.

10. Amal Jubran et al., "Long-term outcome after prolonged mechanical ventilation," *American Journal of Respiratory and Critical Care Medicine* 199, no. 12 (June 2019): 1508.

11. William Meadow et al., "Power and limitations of daily prognostications of death in the medical intensive care unit," *Critical Care Medicine* 39, no. 3 (March 2011): 474.

12. Jason M. Breslow, "Dr. Atul Gawande: 'Hope is not a plan' when doctors, patients talk death," Frontline, pbs.org, accessed February 15, 2021, https://www.pbs.org/wgbh/frontline/article/dr-atul-gawande-hope-is-not-a-plan-when-doctors-patients-talk-death/.

13. Nicholas A. Christakis et al., "Extent and determinants of error in doctors' prognoses in terminally ill patients: Prospective cohort study," *British Medical Journal* 320, no. 7233 (February 2000): 469.

14. Judith E. Nelson et al., "Communication about chronic critical illness," *Archives of Internal Medicine* 167, no. 22 (December 2007): 2509–2515.

15. Lucas S. Zier et al., "Surrogate decision makers' interpretation of prognostic information: A mixed-methods study," *Annals of Internal Medicine* 156, no. 5 (March 2012): 360.

16. Sarah Train et al., "Frightening and traumatic memories early after intensive care discharge," *American Journal of Respiratory and Critical Care Medicine* 199, no. 1 (January 2019): 120.

CHAPTER 7

1. Sarah H. Cross et al., letter to the editor, "Changes in the place of death in the United States," *New England Journal of Medicine* 381, no. 24 (December 2019): 2369.

2. "Organ Donation Statistics," Organdonor.gov, Health Resources and Services Administration, accessed February 15, 2021, https://www.organdonor.gov/statistics -stories/statistics.html.

3. Colin R. Cooke et al., "Predictors of time to death after terminal withdrawal of mechanical ventilation in the ICU," *Chest* 138, no. 2 (August 2010): 289.

4. Bradford Winters et al., "Diagnostic errors in the intensive care unit: A systematic review of autopsy studies," *British Medical Journal* 21, no. 11 (November 2012): 894.

5. Niklas Friberg et al., "Cause of death and significant disease found at autopsy," *Virchows Archiv* 475, no. 6 (November 2019): 781.

CHAPTER 8

1. Mark Unroe et al., "One-year trajectories of care and resource utilization for recipients of prolonged mechanical ventilation: A cohort study," *Annals of Internal Medicine* 153, no. 3 (August 2010): 171.

2. Jeremy M. Kahn et al., "Long-term acute care hospital utilization after critical illness," *Journal of the American Medical Association* 303, no. 22 (June 2010): 2257.

3. Mark E. Mikkelsen et al., "Post-intensive care syndrome (PICS)," UpToDate, accessed February 15, 2021, https://www.uptodate.com/contents/post-intensive-care -syndrome-pics.

4. Robert Hatch et al., "Anxiety, depression, and post-traumatic stress disorder after critical illness: A UK-wide prospective cohort study," *Critical Care* 22, no. 310 (November 2018): https://doi.org/10.1186/s13054-018-2223-6.

5. Dimitry S. Davydow et al., "Psychiatric symptoms and acute care service utilization over the course of the year following medical-surgical intensive care unit admission: A longitudinal investigation," *Critical Care Medicine* 42, no. 12 (December 2014): 2473.

6. Marcus Altman et al., "Sleep disturbance after hospitalization and critical illness: A systematic review," *Annals of the American Thoracic Society* 14, no. 9 (September 2017): 1457.

7. Mark E. Mikkelsen et al., "Post-intensive care syndrome (PICS)," UpToDate, accessed February 15, 2021, https://www.uptodate.com/contents/post-intensive-care -syndrome-pics.

8. David C. Van Pelt et al., "Informal caregiver burden among survivors of prolonged mechanical ventilation," *American Journal of Respiratory and Critical Care Medicine* 175, no. 2 (January 2007): 167.

9. KyungAh Im et al., "Prevalence and outcomes of caregiving after prolonged (≥48 hours) mechanical ventilation in the ICU," *Chest* 125, no. 2 (February 2004): 597.

10. "THRIVE," SCCM.org, Society of Critical Care Medicine, accessed February 15, 2021, https://www.sccm.org/Research/Quality/THRIVE.

11. M. E. Major et al., "Surviving critical illness: What is next? An expert consensus statement on physical rehabilitation after hospital discharge," *Critical Care* 20, no. 1 (October 2016): 354.

12. Brett C. Norman et al., "Employment outcomes after critical illness: An analysis of the bringing to light the risk factors and incidence of neuropsychological dysfunction in ICU survivors cohort," *Critical Care Medicine* 44, no. 11 (November 2016): 2003.

13. Carlos Dobkin, "The economic consequences of hospital admissions," *American Economic Review* 108, no. 2 (February 2018): 308.

14. Nita Khandelwal et al., "Prevalence, risk factors, and outcomes of financial stress in survivors of critical illness," *Critical Care Medicine* 46, no. 6 (June 2018): e530.

15. David U. Himmelstein et al., "Medical bankruptcy: Still common despite the Affordable Care Act," *American Journal of Public Health* 109 (February 2019): 431.

16. "Consumer credit reports: A study of medical and non-medical collections," Files.consumerfinance.gov, Consumer Financial Protection Bureau, accessed February 15, 2021, https://files.consumerfinance.gov/f/201412_cfpb_reports_consumer-credit-medical-and-non-medical-collections.pdf.

17. Gina Martinez, "GoFundMe CEO: One-third of site's donations are to cover medical costs," Time.com, accessed February 15, 2021, https://time.com/5516037/gofundme-medical-bills-one-third-ceo/.

CONCLUSION

1. Cynthia J. Gries et al., "Predictors of symptoms of posttraumatic stress and depression in family members after patient death in the ICU," *Chest* 137, no. 2 (February 2010): 280.

2. Elie Azoulay et al., "Risk of post-traumatic stress symptoms in family members of intensive care unit patients," *American Journal of Respiratory and Critical Care Medicine* 171, no. 9 (May 2005): 987.

3. "Connect with Patients and Families," THRIVE, Society of Critical Care Medicine, SCCM.org, accessed February 15, 2021, https://www.sccm.org/MyICUCare/THRIVE/Connect-With-Patients-and-Families.

Bibliography

Afdhal, Nezam H. "Acalculous cholecystitis: Clinical manifestations, diagnosis, and management." UpToDate. Accessed February 20, 2021. https://www.upto date.com/contents/acalculous-cholecystitis-clinical-manifestations-diagnosis-and -management.

Alper, Eric, Terrence A. O'Malley, and Jeffrey Greenwald. "Hospital discharge and readmission." UpToDate. Accessed February 20, 2021. https://www.uptodate.com/ contents/hospital-discharge-and-readmission.

Altman, Marcus, Melissa P. Knauert, and Margaret A. Pisani. "Sleep disturbance after hospitalization and critical illness: A systematic review." *Annals of the American Thoracic Society* 14, no. 9 (September 2017): 1457–1468.

Andersen, Lars W., Mathias J. Holmberg, Katherine M. Berg, Michael W. Donnino, and Asger Granfeldt. "In-hospital cardiac arrest: A review." *Journal of the American Medical Association* 321, no. 12 (March 2019): 1200–1210.

Anderson, Deverick J., and Daniel J. Sexton. "Overview of control measures for prevention of surgical site infection in adults." UpToDate. Accessed February 20, 2021. https://www.uptodate.com/contents/overview-of-control-measures-for-prevention -of-surgical-site-infection-in-adults.

Anderson, H. Vernon, Richard E. Shaw, Ralph G. Brindis, Kathleen Hewitt, Ronald J. Krone, Peter C. Block, Charles R. McKay, and William S. Weintraub. "A contemporary overview of percutaneous coronary interventions: The American College of Cardiology-National Cardiovascular Data Registry (ACC-NCDR)." *Journal of the American College of Cardiology* 39, no. 7 (April 2002): 1096–1103.

Anesi, George L. "Coronavirus disease 2019 (COVID-19): Critical care and airway management issues." UpToDate. Accessed February 14, 2021. https://

www.uptodate.com/contents/coronavirus-disease-2019-covid-19-critical-care-and
-airway-management-issues.

Angus, Derek C., Amber E. Barnato, Walter T. Linde-Zwirble, Lisa A. Weissfeld, R.
Scott Watson, Tim Rickert, and Gordon D. Rubenfeld. "Use of intensive care at the
end of life in the United States: An epidemiologic study." *Critical Care Medicine* 32,
no. 3 (March 2004): 638–643.

Auld, Sara C., Mark Caridi-Scheible, James M. Blum, Chad Robichaux, Colleen Kraft,
Jesse T. Jacob, Craig S. Jabaley et al. "ICU and ventilator mortality among critically
ill adults with coronavirus disease 2019." *Critical Care Medicine* 48, no. 9 (September 2020): e799–e804.

Azoulay, Elie, Frederic Pochard, Nancy Kentish-Barnes, Sylvie Chevret, Jerome Aboab,
Christophe Adrie, Djilali Annane et al. "Risk of post-traumatic stress symptoms in
family members of intensive care unit patients." *American Journal of Respiratory and
Critical Care Medicine* 171, no. 9 (May 2005): 987–994.

Bartlett, Robert. "Extracorporeal membrane oxygenation (ECMO) in adults." UpTo-
Date. Accessed February 17, 2021. https://www.uptodate.com/contents/extracorpo
real-membrane-oxygenation-ecmo-in-adults.

Beigel, John H., Kay M. Tomashek, Lori E. Dodd, Aneesh K. Mehta, Barry S. Zing-
man, Andre C. Kalil, Elizabeth Hohmann et al. "Remdesivir for the treatment of
Covid-19: Final report." *New England Journal of Medicine* 383, no. 19 (November 2020): 1813–1826.

Berlin, David A., Roy M. Gulik, and Fernando J. Martinez. "Severe Covid-19." *New
England Journal of Medicine* 383, no. 25 (December 2020): 2451–2460.

Bienvenu, Oscar J., Elizabeth Dolantuoni, Pedro A. Mendez-Tellez, Victor D. Dinglas,
Carl Shanholtz, Nadia Husain, Cheryl R. Dennison, Margaret S. Herridge, Peter J.
Pronovost, and Dale M. Needham. "Depressive symptoms and impaired physical
function after acute lung injury: A 2-year longitudinal study." *American Journal of
Respiratory and Critical Care Medicine* 185, no. 5 (March 2012): 517–524.

Breslow, Jason M. "Dr. Atul Gawande: 'Hope is not a plan' when doctors, patients
talk death," Frontline, pbs.org. Accessed February 15, 2021. https://www.pbs.org/
wgbh/frontline/article/dr-atul-gawande-hope-is-not-a-plan-when-doctors-patients
-talk-death/.

Brown, Calvin A. and Sakles, John C. "Rapid sequence intubation for adults outside
the operating room." UpToDate. Accessed February 17, 2021. https://www.uptodate
.com/contents/rapid-sequence-intubation-for-adults-outside-the-operating-room.

Caliendo, Angela M., and Kimberly E. Hanson. "Coronavirus disease 2019 (COVID-
19): Diagnosis." UpToDate. Accessed February 20, 2021. https://www.uptodate
.com/contents/coronavirus-disease-2019-covid-19-diagnosis.

Carrozza, Joseph P. "Complications of diagnostic cardiac catheterization." UpToDate.
Accessed February 2021. https://www.uptodate.com/contents/complications-of
-diagnostic-cardiac-catheterization.

Carrozza, Joseph P., and Thomas Levin. "Periprocedural complications of percutaneous coronary intervention." UpToDate. Accessed February 17, 2021. https://www

.uptodate.com/contents/periprocedural-complications-of-percutaneous-coronary
-intervention.

Carson, Jeffrey L., and Steven Kleinman. "Indications and hemoglobin thresholds for red blood cell transfusion in the adult." UpToDate. Accessed February 17, 2021. https://www.uptodate.com/contents/indications-and-hemoglobin-thresholds-for
-red-blood-cell-transfusion-in-the-adult.

Carson, Shannon S., and Peter B. Bach. "Predicting mortality in patients suffering from prolonged critical illness: An assessment of four severity-of-illness measures." *Chest* 120, no. 3 (September 2001): 928–933.

Cavallazzi, Rodrigo, Mohamed Saad, and Paul E. Marik. "Delirium in the ICU: An overview." *Annals of Intensive Care* 2, no. 1 (December 2012): 49–59.

Centers for Disease Control and Prevention. "Operational considerations for adapting a contact tracing program to respond to the COVID-19 pandemic." CDC.gov. Accessed February 9, 2021. https://www.cdc.gov/coronavirus/2019-ncov/global
-covid-19/operational-considerations-contact-tracing.html#.

Centers for Medicare and Medicaid Services. "Hospital visitation: Phase II visitation for patients who are COVID-19 negative." CMS.gov. Accessed February 9, 2021. https://www.cms.gov/files/document/covid-hospital-visitation-phase-ii-visitation-covid-negative-patients.pdf.

Centers for Medicare and Medicaid Services. "State operations manual, Appendix A: Survey protocol, regulations and interpretive guidelines for hospitals." CMS.gov. Accessed February 9, 2021. https://www.cms.gov/regulations-and-guidance/guid
ance/transmittals/downloads/r75soma.pdf.

Chan, Paul S., Brahmajee K. Nallamothu, Harlan M. Krumholz, John A. Spertus, Yan Li, Bradley G. Hammill, and Lesley H. Curtis. "Long-term outcomes in elderly survivors of in-hospital cardiac arrest." *New England Journal of Medicine* 368, no. 11 (March 2013): 1023–1026.

Chapman, Jason T., Jeff Breeding, Stephen J. Kerr, Marko Bajic, Priya Nair, and Hergen Buscher. "CNS complications in adult patients treated with extracorporeal membrane oxygenation." *Critical Care Medicine* 49, no. 2 (February 2021): 282–291.

Chelluri, Lakshmipathy, Kyung Ah Im, Steven H. Belle, Richard Schulz, Armando J. Rotondi, Michael P. Donahoe, Carl A. Sirio, Aaron B. Mendelsohn, and Michael R. Pinsky. "Long-term mortality and quality of life after prolonged mechanical ventilation." *Critical Care Medicine* 32, no. 1 (January 2004): 61–69.

Cho, Eun, Kyung Jae Lim, Jeong Hyun Jo, Gyoo-Sik Jung, and Byeong Ho Park. "Failed inferior vena cava filter retrieval by conventional method: Analysis of its causes and retrieval of it by modified double-loop technique." *Phlebology* 30, no. 8 (September 2015): 549–556.

Cho, Sung-Min, Abhishek Deshpande, Vinay Pasupuleti, Adrian V. Hernandez, and Ken Uchino. "Radiographic and clinical brain infarcts in cardiac and diagnostic procedures." *Stroke* 48, no. 10 (September 2017): 2753–2759.

Christakis, Nicholas A., and Elizabeth B. Lamont. "Extent and determinants of error in doctors' prognoses in terminally ill patients: Prospective cohort study." *British Medical Journal* 320, no. 7233 (February 2000): 469–473.

Chukmaitov, Askar, Cathy J. Bradley, Bassam Dahman, Umaporn Siangphoe, Joan L. Warren, and Carrie N. Klabunde. "Association of polypectomy techniques, endoscopist volume, and facility type with colonoscopy complications." *Gastrointestinal Endoscopy* 77, no. 3 (March 2013): 436–446.

Cohen, Jonathan, and David A. Greenwald. "Overview of upper gastrointestinal endoscopy (esophagogastroduodenoscopy)." UpToDate. Accessed February 17, 2021. https://www.uptodate.com/contents/overview-of-upper-gastrointestinal-endoscopy -esophagogastroduodenoscopy.

Combes, Alain, Marie-Alyette Costa, Jean-Louis Trouillet, Jerome Baudot, Mourad Mokhtari, Claude Gibert, and Jean Chastre. "Morbidity, mortality, and quality-of -life outcomes of patients requiring > or = 14 days of mechanical ventilation." *Critical Care Medicine* 31, no. 5 (May 2003): 1373–1381.

Consumer Financial Protection Bureau. "Consumer credit reports: A study of medical and non-medical collections." Files.consumerfinance.gov. Accessed February 15, 2021. https://files.consumerfinance.gov/f/201412_cfpb_reports_consumer-credit -medical-and-non-medical-collections.pdf.

Cooke, Colin R., David L. Hotchkin, Ruth A. Engelberg, Lewis Rubinson, and J. Randall Curtis. "Predictors of time to death after terminal withdrawal of mechanical ventilation in the ICU." *Chest* 138, no. 2 (August 2010): 289–297.

Cox, Christopher E., Shannon S. Carson, Jennifer H. Lindquist, Maren K. Olsen, Joseph A. Govert, and Lakshmipathy Chelluri. "Differences in one-year health outcomes and resource utilization by definition of prolonged mechanical ventilation: A prospective cohort study." *Critical Care* 11, no. 1 (January 2007): https:// doi.org/10.1186/cc5667.

Cox, Christopher E., Tereza Martinu, Shailaja J. Sathy, Alison S. Clay, Jessica Chia, Alice L. Gray, Maren K. Olsen, Joseph A. Govert, Shannon S. Carson, and James A. Tulsky. "Expectations and outcomes of prolonged mechanical ventilation." *Critical Care Medicine* 37, no. 11 (November 2009): 2888–2894.

Cross, Sarah H., and Haider J. Warraich. Letter to the editor. "Changes in the place of death in the United States." *New England Journal of Medicine* 381, no. 24 (December 2019): 2369–2370.

Cuker, Adam, and Flora Peyvandi. "Coronavirus disease 2019 (COVID-19): Hypercoagulability." UpToDate. Accessed February 14, 2021. https://www.uptodate.com/ contents/coronavirus-disease-2019-covid-19-hypercoagulability.

Cummings, Matthew J., Matthew R. Baldwin, Darryl Abrams, Samuel D. Jacobson, Benjamin J. Meyer, Elizabeth M. Balough, Justin G. Aaron et al. "Epidemiology, clinical course, and outcomes of critically ill adults with COVID-19 in New York City: A prospective cohort study." *Lancet* 395, no. 10239 (June 2020): 1763–1770.

Damuth, Emily, Jessica A. Mitchell, Jason L. Bartock, Brian W. Roberts, and Tephen Trzeciak. "Long-term survival of critically ill patients treated with prolonged mechanical ventilation: A systematic review and meta-analysis." *Lancet Respiratory Medicine* 3, no. 7 (July 2015): 544–553.

Davydow, Dimitry S., Catherine L. Hough, Douglas Zatzick, and Wayne J. Katon. "Psychiatric symptoms and acute care service utilization over the course of the year following medical-surgical intensive care unit admission: A longitudinal investigation." *Critical Care Medicine* 42, no. 12 (December 2014): 2473–2481.

De Jonghe, Bernard, Tarek Sharshar, Jean-Pascal Lefaucheur, Francois-Jerome Authier, Isabelle Durand-Zaleski, Mohamed Boussarsar, Charles Cerf et al. "Paresis acquired in the intensive care unit: A prospective multicenter study." *Journal of the American Medical Association* 288, no. 22 (December 2002): 2859–2867.

DeLegge, Mark H. "Gastrostomy Tubes: Complications and Their Management." UpToDate. Accessed February 17, 2021. https://www.uptodate.com/contents/gastrostomy-tubes-complications-and-their-management.

Dinglas, Victor D., Lisa Aronson Friedman, Elizabeth Colantuoni, Pedro A. Mendez-Tellez, Carl B. Shanholtz, Nancy D. Ciesla, Peter J. Pronovost, and Dale M. Needham. "Muscle weakness and 5-year survival in acute respiratory distress syndrome survivors." *Critical Care Medicine* 45, no. 3 (March 2017): 446–453.

Dobkin, Carlos, Amy Finkelstein, Raymond Kluender, and Matthew J. Notowidigdo. "The economic consequences of hospital admissions." *American Economic Review* 108, no. 2 (February 2018): 308–352.

Esteban, Andres, Antonio Anzueto, Fernando Frutos, Inmaculada Alia, Laurent Brochard, Thomas E. Stewart, Salvador Benito et al. "Characteristics and outcomes in adult patients receiving mechanical ventilation: A 28-day international study." *Journal of the American Medical Association* 287, no. 3 (January 2002): 345–355.

Fan, Eddy, Jeremy R. Beitler, Laurent Brochard, Carolyn S. Calfee, Niall D. Ferguson, Arthur S. Slutsky, and Daniel Brodie. "COVID-19 associated acute respiratory distress syndrome: Is a different approach to management warranted?" *Lancet Respiratory Medicine* 8, no. 8 (August 2020): 816–821.

Fedullo, Peter F., and Anne Roberts. "Placement of vena cava filters and their complications." UpToDate. Accessed February 17, 2021. https://www.uptodate.com/contents/placement-of-vena-cava-filters-and-their-complications.

Ferguson, James J., Marc Cohen, Robert J. Freedman Jr., Gregg W. Stone, Michael F. Miller, Debra L. Joseph, and E. Magnus Ohman. "The current practice of intra-aortic balloon counterpulsation: Results from the Benchmark Registry." *Journal of the American College of Cardiology* 38, no. 5 (November 2001): 1456–1462.

Ferrando, Carlos, Fernando Suarez-Sipmann, Ricard Mellado-Artigas, Maria Hernandez, Alfredo Gea, Egoitz Arruti, Cesar Aldecoa et al. "Clinical features, ventilatory management, and outcome of ARDS caused by COVID-19 are similar to other causes of ARDS." *Intensive Care Medicine* 46, no. 12 (December 2020): 2200–2211.

Ferreira, Flavio Lopes, Daliana Peres Bota, and Annette Bross. "Serial evaluation of the SOFA score to predict outcome in critically ill patients." *Journal of the American Medical Association* 286, no. 14 (October 2001): 1754–1758.

Francis, Joseph, Jr. "Delirium and acute confusional states: Prevention, treatment, and prognosis." UpToDate. Accessed February 20, 2021. https://www.uptodate

.com/contents/delirium-and-acute-confusional-states-prevention-treatment-and -prognosis.

Friberg, Niklas, Oscar Ljungberg, Erik Berglund, David Berglund, Richard Ljungberg, Irina Alafuzoff, and Elisabet Englund. "Cause of death and significant disease found at autopsy." *Virchows Archiv* 475, no. 6 (November 2019): 781–788.

Gawande, Atul. *Being mortal: Medicine and what matters in the end.* New York: Metropolitan Books and Henry Holt and Company, 2014.

Gilman, Matlin, E. Kathleen Adams, Jason M. Hockenberry, Arnold S. Milstein, Ira B. Wilson, and Edmund R. Becker. "Safety-net hospitals more likely than other hospitals to fare poorly under Medicare's Value-Based Purchasing." *Health Affairs* 34, no. 3 (March 2015): 398–405.

Girard, Timothy D., John P. Kress, Barry D. Fuchs, Jason W. W. Thomason, William D. Schweickert, Brenda T. Pun, Darren B. Taichman et al. "Efficacy and safety of a paired sedation and ventilator weaning protocol for mechanically ventilated patients in intensive care (Awakening and Breathing Controlled trial): A randomized controlled trial." *Lancet* 371, no. 9607 (January 2008): 126–134.

Giustino, Gennaro, Sean P. Pinney, Anuradha Lala, Vivek Y. Reddy, Hillary A. Johnston-Cox, Jeffrey I. Mechanick, Jonathan L. Halpern, and Valentin Fuster. "Coronavirus and cardiovascular disease, myocardial injury, and arrhythmia." *Journal of the American College of Cardiology* 76, no. 17 (October 2020): 2011–2023.

Gries, Cynthia J., Ruth A. Engelberg, Erin K. Kross, Doug Zatzick, Elizabeth L. Nielsen, Lois Downey, and J. Randall Curtis. "Predictors of symptoms of posttraumatic stress and depression in family members after patient death in the ICU." *Chest* 137, no. 2 (February 2010): 280–287.

Hale, Conor. "New MIT study puts clinical research success rate at 14 percent." CenterWatch. Accessed February 16, 2021. https://www.centerwatch.com/ articles/12702-new-mit-study-puts-clinical-research-success-rate-at-14-percent.

Han, MeiLan King. "Management and prognosis of patients requiring prolonged mechanical ventilation." UpToDate. Accessed February 15, 2021. https://www.upto date.com/contents/management-and-prognosis-of-patients-requiring-prolonged -mechanical-ventilation.

Hariri, Lida P., Crystal M. North, Angela R. Shih, Rebecca A. Israel, Jason H. Maley, Julian A. Villalba, Vladimir Vinarsky et al. "Lung histopathology in coronavirus disease 2019 as compared with severe acute respiratory syndrome and H1N1 influenza: A systematic review." *Chest* 159, no. 1 (January 2021): 73–84.

Hatch, Robert, Duncan Young, Vicki Barber, John Griffiths, David A. Harrison, and Peter Watkinson. "Anxiety, depression, and post-traumatic stress disorder after critical illness: A UK-wide prospective cohort study." *Critical Care* 22, no. 310 (November 2018): https://doi.org/10.1186/s13054-018-2223-6.

Haudebourg, Anne-Fleur, Francois Perier, Samuel Tuffet, Nicolas de Prost, Keyvan Razazi, Mekonstso Dessap, and Guillaume Carteaux. "Respiratory mechanics of COVID-19- versus non-COVID-19-associated respiratory distress syndrome." *American Journal of Respiratory and Critical Care Medicine* 202, no. 2 (July 2020): 287–290.

Health Resources and Services Administration. "Organ donation statistics." Organdonor.gov. Accessed February 15, 2021. https://www.organdonor.gov/statistics-stories/statistics.html.

Heffner, John E., and Paul Mayo. "Ultrasound-guided thoracentesis." UpToDate. Accessed February 17, 2021. https://www.uptodate.com/contents/ultrasound-guided-thoracentesis.

Herridge, Margaret S., Catherine M. Taney, Andrea Matte, George Tomlinson, Natalia Diaz-Granados, Andrew Cooper, Cameron B. Guest et al. "Functional disability 5 years after acute respiratory distress syndrome." *New England Journal of Medicine* 364, no. 14 (April 2011): 1293–1304.

Himmelstein, David U., Robert M. Lawless, Deborah Thorne, Pamela Foohey, and Steffie Woolhandler. "Medical bankruptcy: Still common despite the Affordable Care Act." *American Journal of Public Health* 109 (February 2019): 431–433.

Hirlekar, G., T. Karlsson, S. Aune, A. Ravn-Fischer, P. Albertsson, J. Herlitz, and B. Libungan. "Survival and neurological outcome in the elderly after in-hospital cardiac arrest." *Resuscitation* 118 (September 2017): 101–106.

Holley, Jean L. "Acute complications during hemodialysis." UpToDate. Accessed February 17, 2021. https://www.uptodate.com/contents/acute-complications-during-hemodialysis.

Hornby, Peter, Wei Shen Lim, Jonathan R. Emberson, Marion Mafham, Jennifer L. Bell, Louise Linsell, Natalie Staplin et al. "Dexamethasone in hospitalized patients with Covid-19: preliminary report." *New England Journal of Medicine*, published ahead of print, July 17, 2020, https://doi.org/10.1056/NEJMoa2021436.

Hosey, Megan M., and Dale M. Needham. "Survivorship after COVID-19 ICU stay." *Nature Reviews Disease Primers* 6, no. 1 (July 2020): 60–61.

Huang, Chaolin, Lixue Huang, Yeming Wang, Xia Li, Lili Ren, Xiaoying Gu, Liang Kang et al. "6-month consequences of COVID-19 in patients discharged from hospital: A cohort study." *Lancet* 397, no. 10270 (January 2021): 220–232.

Huggins, John T., Shamus R. Carr, and George A. Woodward. "Thoracostomy tubes and catheters: Placement techniques and complications." UpToDate. Accessed February 17, 2021. https://www.uptodate.com/contents/thoracostomy-tubes-and-catheters-placement-techniques-and-complications.

Huggins, John T., and Amit Chopra. "Large volume (therapeutic) thoracentesis: procedure and complications." UpToDate. Accessed February 17, 2021. https://www.uptodate.com/contents/large-volume-therapeutic-thoracentesis-procedure-and-complications.

Hyzy, Robert C. "Complications of the endotracheal tube following initial placement: Prevention and management in adult intensive care unit patients." UpToDate. Accessed February 20, 2021. https://www.uptodate.com/contents/complications-of-the-endotracheal-tube-following-initial-placement-prevention-and-management-in-adult-intensive-care-unit-patients.

Hyzy, Robert C., and Jakob I. McSparron. "Overview of tracheostomy." UpToDate. Accessed February 17, 2021. https://www.uptodate.com/contents/overview-of-tracheostomy.

Im, KyungAh, Steven H. Belle, Richard Schulz, Aaron B. Mendelsohn, and Laksh-mipathi Chelluri. "Prevalence and outcomes of caregiving after prolonged (≥48 hours) mechanical ventilation in the ICU." *Chest* 125, no. 2 (February 2004): 597–606.

Islam, Shaheen. "Flexible bronchoscopy in adults: Preparation, procedural technique, and complications." UpToDate. Accessed February 17, 2021. https://www.uptodate .com/contents/flexible-bronchoscopy-in-adults-preparation-procedural-technique -and-complications.

Iwashyna, Theodore J., Jason D. Christie, Jeremy M. Kahn, and David A. Asch. "Uncharted paths: Hospital networks in critical care." *Chest* 135, no. 3 (March 2009): 828–833.

Jabre, Patricia, Vanessa Belpomme, Elie Azoulay, Line Jacob, Lionel Bertrand, Frederic Lapostolle, Karim Tazarourte et al. "Family presence during cardiopulmonary resuscitation." *New England Journal of Medicine* 368, no. 11 (March 2013): 1008–1018.

Jacob, Jesse T., and Robert Gaynes. "Intravascular catheter-related infection: Prevention." UpToDate. Accessed Febrary 20, 2021. https://www.uptodate.com/contents/intravascular-catheter-related-infection-prevention.

Jain, Prasoon, Jorge P. Parada, and Annette David. "Overuse of the indwelling urinary tract catheter in hospitalized medical patients." *Archives of Internal Medicine* 155, no. 13 (July 1995): 1425–1429.

Jubran, Amal, Brydon J. B. Grant, Lisa A. Duffner, Eileen G. Collins, Dorothy M. Lanuza, Leslie A. Hoffman, and Martin J. Tobin. "Long-term outcome after prolonged mechanical ventilation." *American Journal of Respiratory and Critical Care Medicine* 199, no. 12 (June 2019): 1508–1516.

Kahn, Jeremy M., Nicole M. Benson, Dina Appleby, Shannon S. Carson, and Theodore J. Iwashyna. "Long-term acute care hospital utilization after critical illness." *Journal of the American Medical Association* 303, no. 22 (June 2010): 2253–2259.

Kearney, Thomas J., and Michael M. Shabot. "Pulmonary artery rupture associated with the Swan-Ganz catheter." *Chest* 108, no. 5 (November 1995): 1349–1352.

Khandelwal, Nita, Catherine L. Hough, Lois Downey, Ruth A. Engelberg, Shannon S. Carson, Douglas B. White, Jeremy M. Kahn et al. "Prevalence, risk factors, and outcomes of financial stress in survivors of critical illness." *Critical Care Medicine* 46, no. 6 (June 2018): e530–e539.

Kross, Erin K., Ruth A. Engleberg, Cynthia J. Gries, Elizabeth L. Nielsen, Douglas Zatzick, and J. Randall Curtis. "ICU care associated with symptoms of depression and posttraumatic stress disorder among family members of patients who die in the ICU." *Chest* 139, no. 4 (April 2011): 795–801.

Lacomis, David. "Neuromuscular weakness related to critical illness." UpToDate. Accessed February 20, 2021. https://www.uptodate.com/contents/neuromuscular-weakness-related-to-critical-illness.

Ladopoulos, Theodoros, Marcia Giannaki, Christina Alexopoulou, Athanasia Proklou, Emmanuel Pediaditis, and Eumorfia Kondili. "Gastrointestinal dysmotility in critically ill patients." *Annals of Gastroenterology* 31, no. 3 (March 2018): 1–9.

Laham, Roger J., and Duane S. Pinto. "Intraaortic balloon pump counterpulsation." UpToDate. Accessed February 17, 2021. https://www.uptodate.com/contents/intraaortic-balloon-pump-counterpulsation.

Lamont, J. Thomas, Johan S. Bakken, and Ciaran P. Kelly. "Clostridioides difficile infection in adults: Epidemiology, microbiology, and pathophysiology." UpToDate. Accessed February 20, 2021. https://www.uptodate.com/contents/clostridioides-formerly-clostridium-difficile-infection-in-adults-epidemiology-microbiology-and-pathophysiology.

Law, Anica C., Jennifer P. Stevens, and Allan J. Walkey. "Gastrostomy tube use in the critically ill, 1994–2014." *Annals of the American Thoracic Society* 16, no. 6 (June 2019): 724–730.

Leape, Lucian L., Troyen A. Brennan, Nan Laird, Ann G. Lawthers, A. Russell Localio, Benjamin A. Barnes, Liesi Hebert, Joseph P. Newhouse, Paul C. Weiler, and Howard Hiatt. "The nature of adverse events in hospitalized patients: Results of the Harvard Medical Practice Study II." *New England Journal of Medicine* 324, no. 6 (February 1991): 377–384.

Lee, Linda, and John R. Saltzman. "Overview of colonoscopy in adults." UpToDate. Accessed February 17, 2021. https://www.uptodate.com/contents/overview-of-colonoscopy-in-adults.

Leisman, Daniel E., Lukas Ronner, Rachel Pinotti, Matthew D. Taylor, Pratik Sinha, Carolyn S. Calfee, Alexandre V. Hirayama et al. "Cytokine elevation in severe and critical COVID-19: A rapid systematic review, meta-analysis, and comparison with other inflammatory syndromes." *Lancet Respiratory Medicine* 8, no. 12 (December 2020): 1233–1244.

Leung, Lawrence L. K. "Disseminated intravascular coagulation: Evaluation and management." UpToDate. Accessed February 22, 2021. https://www.uptodate.com/contents/disseminated-intravascular-coagulation-dic-in-adults-evaluation-and-management.

Lighthall, Geoffrey, and Luis Verduzco. "Survival after long-term residence in an intensive care unit." *Federal Practitioner* 33, no. 6 (June 2016): 18–27.

Loser, Chr., G. Aschl, X. Hebuterne, E. M. H. Mathus-Vliegen, M. Muscaritoli, Y. Niv, H. Rollins, P. Singer, and R. H. Skelly. "ESPEN guidelines on artificial enteral nutrition: Percutaneous endoscopic gastrostomy." *Clinical Nutrition* 24, no. 5 (October 2005): 848–861.

Mackey, Katherine, Chelsea K. Ayers, Karli K. Kondo, Somnath Saha, Shailesh M. Advani, Sarah Young, Hunter Spencer, Max Rusek, Johanna Anderson, Stephanie Veazie, Mia Smith, and Devan Kansagara. "Racial and ethnic disparities in COVID-19-related infections, hospitalizations, and deaths." *Annals of Internal Medicine*, published ahead of print, December 1, 2020. https://doi.org/10.7326/M20-6306.

Major, M. E., R. Kwakman, M. E. Kho, B. Connolly, D. McWilliams, L. Denehy, S. Hanekom et al. "Surviving critical illness: What is next? An expert consensus statement on physical rehabilitation after hospital discharge." *Critical Care* 20, no. 1 (October 2016): 354–364.

Malhotra, Atul, and Robert M. Kacmarek. "Prone ventilation for adult patients with acute respiratory distress syndrome." UpToDate. Accessed February 9, 2021. https://www.uptodate.com/contents/prone-ventilation-for-adult-patients-with-acute-respiratory-distress-syndrome.

Manara, A. R., J. A. L. Pittman, and F. E. M. Braddon. "Reasons for withdrawing treatment in patients receiving intensive care." *Anaesthesia* 53, no. 6 (June 1998): 523–528.

Marchaim, Dror, and Keith Kaye. "Infections and antimicrobial resistance in the intensive care unit: Epidemiology and prevention." UpToDate. Accessed February 20, 2021. https://www.uptodate.com/contents/infections-and-antimicrobial-resistance-in-the-intensive-care-unit-epidemiology-and-prevention.

Marino, Paul L. *The ICU Book*. 4th ed. Philadelphia: Wolters Kluwer Health/Lippincott Williams & Wilkins, 2014.

Marklin, Gary F., and Ron Shapiro. "Evaluation of the potential deceased organ donor." UpToDate. Accessed February 22, 2021. https://www.uptodate.com/contents/evaluation-of-the-potential-deceased-organ-donor-adult.

Martinez, Gina. "GoFundMe CEO: One-third of site's donations are to cover medical costs." U.S. Healthcare, Time.com. Accessed February 15, 2021. https://time.com/5516037/gofundme-medical-bills-one-third-ceo/.

Mateen, Farrah J., Rajanandini Mralidharan, Russell T. Shinohara, Joseph E. Parisi, Gregory J. Schears, and Eelco F. M. Wijdicks. "Neurological injury in adults treated with extracorporeal membrane oxygenation." *Archives of Neurology* 68, no. 12 (December 2011): 1543–1549.

McAdam, Jennifer L., Kathleen A. Dracup, Douglas B. White, Dorothy K. Fontaine, and Kathleen A. Puntillo. "Symptom experiences of family members of intensive care unit patients at high risk for dying." *Critical Care Medicine* 38, no. 4 (April 2010): 1078–1085.

McIntosh, Kenneth. "Coronavirus disease 2019 (COVID-19): Clinical features." UpToDate. Accessed February 20, 2021. https://www.uptodate.com/contents/coronavirus-disease-2019-covid-19-clinical-features.

McIntosh, Kenneth. "Coronavirus disease 2019 (COVID-19): Epidemiology, virology, and prevention." UpToDate. Accessed February 20, 2021. https://www.uptodate.com/contents/coronavirus-disease-2019-covid-19-epidemiology-virology-and-prevention.

Meadow, William, Anne Pohlman, Laura Frain, Yaya Ren, John P. Kress, Winnie Teuteberg, and Jesse Hall. "Power and limitations of daily prognostications of death in the medical intensive care unit." *Critical Care Medicine* 39, no. 3 (March 2011): 474–479.

Medpage Today. "Trials halt full-dose clot prophylaxix for severe COVID-19." Accessed February 14, 2021. https://www.medpagetoday.com/infectiousdisease/covid19/90351.

Meyerowitz-Katz, Gideon, and Lea Merone. "A systematic review and meta-analysis of published research data on COVID-19 infection fatality rates." *International Journal of Infectious Diseases*. Published ahead of print, September 29, 2020. https://doi.org/10.1016/j.ijid.2020.09.1464.

Mikkelsen, Mark E., Giora Netzer, and Theodore Iwashyna. "Post-intensive care syndrome (PICS)." UpToDate. Accessed February 15, 2021. https://www.uptodate .com/contents/post-intensive-care-syndrome-pics.

Mikkelsen, Mark E., Jason D. Christie, Paul N. Lanken, Rosette C. Biester, B. Taylor Thompson, Scarlett L. Bellamy, A. Russell Localio, Ejigayehu Demissie, Ramona O. Hopkins, and Derek C. Angus. "The adult respiratory distress syndrome cognitive outcomes study: Long-term neuropsychological function in survivors of acute lung injury." *American Journal of Respiratory and Critical Care Medicine* 185, no. 12 (June 2012): 1307–1315.

Moitra, Vivek K., Carmen Guerra, Walter T. Linde-Zwirble, and Hannah Wunsch. "Relationship between ICU length of stay and long-term mortality for elderly ICU survivors." *Critical Care Medicine* 44, no. 4 (April 2016): 655–662.

Nelson, Judith E., Alice F. Mercado, Sharon L. Camhi, Nidhi Tandon, Sylvan Wallenstein, Gary I. August, and Sean Morrison. "Communication about chronic critical illness." *Archives of Internal Medicine* 167, no. 22 (December 2007): 2509–2515.

Neviere, Remi. "Sepsis syndromes in adults: Epidemiology, presentation, diagnosis, and prognosis." UpToDate. Accessed February 22, 2021. https://www.uptodate.com/ contents/sepsis-syndromes-in-adults-epidemiology-definitions-clinical-presentation -diagnosis-and-prognosis.

Norman, Brett C., James C. Jackson, John A. Graves, Timothy D. Girard, Pratik Pandharipande, Nathan Brummel, Li Wang, Jennifer L. Thompson, Rameela Chandrasekhar, and E. Wesley Ely. "Employment outcomes after critical illness: An analysis of the bringing to light the risk factors and incidence of neuropsychological dysfunction in ICU survivors cohort." *Critical Care Medicine* 44, no. 11 (November 2016): 2003–2009.

Palmore, Tara N. "Coronavirus disease 2019 (COVID-19): Infection control in health care and home settings." UpToDate. Accessed February 20, 2021. https://www .uptodate.com/contents/coronavirus-disease-2019-covid-19-infection-control-in -health-care-and-home-settings.

Parasher, Anant. "COVID-19: Current understanding of its pathophysiology, clinical presentation and treatment." *Postgraduate Medical Journal.* Published ahead of print, September 25, 2020. https://doi.org/10.1136/postgradmedj-2020-138577.

Prescott, Hallie C., and Timothy D. Girard. "Recovery from severe COVID-19: Leveraging the lessons of survival from sepsis." *Journal of the American Medical Association* 324, no. 8 (August 2020): 739–740.

Runyon, Bruce A. "Diagnostic and therapeutic abdominal paracentesis." UpToDate. Accessed February 17, 2021. https://www.uptodate.com/contents/ diagnostic-and-therapeutic-abdominal-paracentesis.

Sakr, Yasser, Cora L. Moreira, Andrew Rhodes, Niall D. Ferguson, Ruth Kleinpell, Peter Pickkers, Michael A. Kuiper, Jeffrey Lipman, and Jean-Louis Vincent. "The impact of hospital and ICU organizational factors on outcome in critically ill patients: Results from the extended prevalence of infection in intensive care study." *Critical Care Medicine* 43, no. 3 (March 2015): 519–526.

Scalise, Paul, Steven R. Prunk, Dave Healy, and John Votto. "The incidence of tracheo-arterial fistula in patients with chronic tracheostomy tubes: A retrospective study of 544 patients in a long-term care facility." *Chest* 128, no. 6 (December 2005): 3906–3909.

Scheinhorn, David J., Meg Stearn Hassenpflug, John J. Votto, David C. Chao, Scott K. Epstein, Gordon S. Doig, E. Bert Knight, and Richard A. Petrak. "Post-ICU mechanical ventilation at 23 long-term care centers: A multicenter outcomes study." *Chest* 131, no. 1 (January 2007): 85–93.

Seres, David. "Nutrition support in critically ill patients: An overview." UpToDate. Accessed February 20, 2021. https://www.uptodate.com/contents/nutrition-support-in-critically-ill-patients-an-overview.

Sidiqui, Haziq. "To suffer alone: Hospital visitation policies during COVID-19." *Journal of Hospital Medicine* 15, no. 11 (November 2020): 694–695.

Siemieniuk, Reed, et al. "Drug treatments for covid-19: Living systematic review and network meta-analysis." *British Medical Journal*. Published ahead of print, July 30, 2020. https://doi.org/10.1136/bmj.m2980.

Siegel, Mark D., Polly E. Parsons, and Geraldine Finlay. "Acute respiratory distress syndrome: Prognosis and outcomes in adults." UpToDate. Accessed February 15, 2021. https://www.uptodate.com/contents/acute-respiratory-distress-syndrome-prognosis-and-outcomes-in-adults.

Silvergleid, Arthur J. "Immunologic transfusion reactions." UpToDate. Accessed February 17, 2021. https://www.uptodate.com/contents/immunologic-transfusion-reactions.

Silvis, Stephen E., Otto Nebel, and Gerald Rogers. "Endoscopic complications: Results of the 1974 American Society for Gastrointestinal Endoscopy Survey." *Journal of the American Medical Association* 235, no. 9 (March 1976): 928–930.

Singh, Jeffrey M., Russell D. MacDonald, and Mahvareh Ahghari. "Critical events during land-based interfacility transport." *Annals of Emergency Medicine* 64, no. 1 (July 2014): 9–15.

Smith, Edward R., and Spideh Amin-Hanjani. "Evaluation and management of elevated intracranial pressure in adults." UpToDate. Accessed February 17, 2021. https://www.uptodate.com/contents/evaluation-and-management-of-elevated-intracranial-pressure-in-adults.

Society for Hospital Epidemiology of America, Association for Practitioners in Infection Control, Centers for Disease Control, and Surgical Infection Society. "Consensus paper on the surveillance of surgical wound infections." *Infection Control and Hospital Epidemiology* 13, no. 10 (October 1992): 599–605.

Society of Critical Care Medicine. "Critical Care Statistics." SCCM.org. Accessed February 15, 2021. https://www.sccm.org/Communications/Critical-Care-Statistics.

Society of Critical Care Medicine. "THRIVE." SCCM.org. Accessed February 15, 2021. https://www.sccm.org/MyICUCare/THRIVE.

Theodore, Arthur C., Gilles Clermont, and Allison Dalton. "Intra-arterial catheterization for invasive monitoring: Indications, insertion techniques, and interpretation." UpToDate. Accessed February 17, 2021. https://www.uptodate.com/contents/intra

-arterial-catheterization-for-invasive-monitoring-indications-insertion-techniques
-and-interpretation.

Tjong, F. V. Y., U. W. de Ruijter, N. E. G. Beurskens, and R. E. Knops. "A comprehensive scoping review on transvenous temporary pacing therapy." *Netherlands Heart Journal* 27 (August 2019): 462–473.

Train, Sarah, Kalliopi Kydonaki, Janice Rattray, Jacqueline Stephen, Christopher J. Weir, and Timothy S. Walsh. "Frightening and traumatic memories early after intensive care discharge." *American Journal of Respiratory and Critical Care Medicine* 199, no. 1 (January 2019): 120–123.

Unger, Joseph M., William E. Barlow, Scott D. Ramsey, Michael LeBlanc, Charles D. Blanke, and Dawn L. Hershman. "The scientific impact of positive and negative phase III cancer clinical trials." *Journal of the American Medical Association Oncology* 2, no. 7 (July 2016): 875–881.

Unroe, Mark, Jeremy M. Kahn, Shannon S. Carson, Joseph A. Govert, Tereza Martinu, Shailaja J. Sathy, Alison S. Clay et al. "One-year trajectories of care and resource utilization for recipients of prolonged mechanical ventilation: A cohort study." *Annals of Internal Medicine* 153, no. 3 (August 2010): 167–175.

Vahidy, Farhaan S., Ashley L. Drews, Faisal N. Masud, Roberta L. Schwartz, Belimat Billy Askary, Marc L. Bloom, and Robert A. Phillips. "Characteristics and outcomes of COVID-19 patients during initial peak and resurgence in the Houston metropolitan area." *Journal of the American Medical Association* 324, no. 10 (September 2020): 998–1000.

Van Pelt, David C., Eric B. Milbrandt, Li Qin, Lisa A. Weissfeld, Armando J. Rotondi, Richard Schulz, Lakshmipathi Chelluri, Derek C. Angus, and Michael R. Pinsky. "Informal caregiver burden among survivors of prolonged mechanical ventilation." *American Journal of Respiratory and Critical Care Medicine* 175, no. 2 (January 2007): 167–173.

Weinhouse, Gerald L. "Pulmonary artery catheterization: Indications, contraindications, and complications in adults." UpToDate. Accessed February 17, 2021. https://www.uptodate.com/contents/pulmonary-artery-catheterization-indications
-contraindications-and-complications-in-adults.

White, Douglas B. "Ethics in the intensive care unit: Informed consent." UpToDate. Accessed February 20, 2021. https://www.uptodate.com/contents/ethics-in-the
-intensive-care-unit-informed-consent.

White, Douglas B. "Withholding and withdrawing ventilatory support in adults in the intensive care unit." UpToDate. Accessed February 20, 2021. https://www.uptodate
.com/contents/withholding-and-withdrawing-ventilatory-support-in-adults-in-the
-intensive-care-unit.

Winters, Bradford, Jason Custer, Samuel M. Galvagno Jr., Elizabeth Colantuoni, Shruti G. Kapoor, Heewon Lee, Victoria Goode et al. "Diagnostic errors in the intensive care unit: A systematic review of autopsy studies." *British Medical Journal* 21, no. 11 (November 2012): 894–902.

Young, Michael P., and Theodore H. Yuo. "Overview of complications of central venous catheters and their prevention." UpToDate. Accessed February 17, 2021.

https://www.uptodate.com/contents/overview-of-complications-of-central-venous
-catheters-and-their-prevention.

Zhao, Zhongyi, Yinhao Wei, and Chuanmin Tao. "An enlightening role for cytokine storm in coronavirus infection." *Clinical Immunology* 222 (January 2021): https:// doi.org/10.1016/j.clim.2020.108615.

Zias, Nikolaos, Alexandra Chroneou, Maher K. Tabba, Anne V. Gonzalez, Anthony W. Gray, Carla R. Lamb, David R. Riker, and John F. Beamis Jr. "Post tracheostomy and post intubation tracheal stenosis: Report of 31 cases and review of the literature." *BMC Pulmonary Medicine* 8, no. 18 (September 2008): 18–27.

Zier, Lucas S., Peter D. Sottile, Seo Yeon Hong, Lisa A. Weissfield, and Douglas B. White. "Surrogate decision makers' interpretation of prognostic information: A mixed-methods study." *Annals of Internal Medicine* 156, no. 5 (March 2012): 360–366.

Zopf, Y., P. Konturek, A. Nuernberger, J. Maiss, J. Zenk, H. Iro, E. G. Hahn, and D. Schwab. "Local infection after placement of percutaneous endoscopic gastrostomy tubes: A prospective study evaluating risk factors." *Canadian Journal of Gastroenterology* 22, no. 12 (December 2008): 987.

Index

Page references for figures are italicized. Acronyms that are used particularly commonly in the ICU are included in the index.

211

About the Author

Dr. Lara Goitein is a Harvard-trained physician specializing in pulmonary and critical care medicine who has worked as a doctor in intensive care units for 12 years. Currently she is President-Elect of Medical Staff at Christus St. Vincent Regional Medical Center in Santa Fe, New Mexico, and founding medical director of a hospital quality program called Clinician-Directed Performance Improvement. She is on the editorial board and is a frequent writer for the medical journal *JAMA Internal Medicine*, and is a reviewer for its series "Physician Work Environment and Well-Being." Dr. Goitein also writes for the lay press, including an article in the *New York Review of Books* called, "Training Young Doctors: The Current Crisis." Her professional interests include measuring and improving healthcare quality, physicians' professional well-being, graduate medical education, the effects of the financial environment on the teaching and practice of medicine, and care at the end of life. She is a graduate of the Intermountain Advanced Training Program in Healthcare Delivery Improvement. Dr. Goitein's work in quality improvement at Christus St. Vincent Regional Medical Center has received national attention: she was a speaker at the IHI/NPSF Patient Safety Congress in Boston in May of 2018, and recently wrote an article about the quality improvement program she directed in *Health Affairs*. Right now, Dr. Goitein is taking a break from clinical practice, and is home with her two sons while they do online school, in Santa Fe, New Mexico.

CPSIA information can be obtained
at www.ICGtesting.com
Printed in the USA
BVHW011938210122
626807BV00002B/117